I0701502

HEALTHY COOKING FOR STROKE PATIENTS

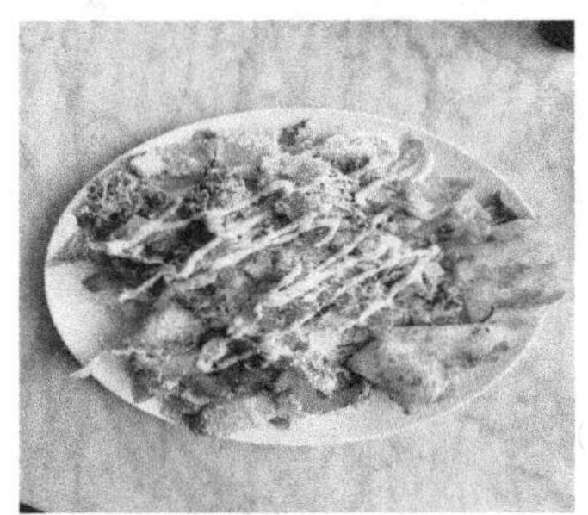

Delicious Recipes and Nutritional Guidance for Stroke Recovery and Heart Health

By

Molly O.harper

Copyright © by Molly O. Harper 2024

All rights reserved.
Before this document is duplicated or reproduced in any manner, the publisher's consent must be gained. Therefore, the contents within can neither be stored electronically, transferred, nor kept in a database. Neither in Part nor full can the document be copied, scanned, faxed, or retained without approval from the publisher or creator.

Table of content

About the book

"Healthy Cooking for Stroke Patients" is a comprehensive guide designed to support stroke survivors in their recovery journey through nutritious and delicious meals. This book offers a wide variety of recipes tailored to meet the specific dietary needs of stroke patients, emphasizing heart-healthy ingredients and easy-to-follow instructions. With expert tips on meal planning, portion control, and cooking techniques, it empowers patients and caregivers alike to create balanced, flavorful dishes that promote healing and overall well-being. Whether you're new to the kitchen or a seasoned cook, "Healthy Cooking for Stroke Patients" provides invaluable resources to make every meal a step towards better health.

Introduction

Recovering from a stroke is a challenging journey that requires not only medical treatment but also a significant lifestyle adjustment, particularly in terms of diet. "Healthy Cooking for Stroke Patients" is an essential guide designed to make this transition smoother and more enjoyable. This book provides a comprehensive collection of recipes that are both delicious and specifically tailored to meet the unique nutritional needs of stroke survivors. Each recipe emphasizes heart-healthy ingredients, mindful preparation, and balanced nutrition, ensuring that every meal supports recovery and overall well-being.

The importance of diet in stroke recovery cannot be overstated. Proper nutrition plays a crucial role in rebuilding strength, reducing the risk of further complications, and promoting overall health. "Healthy Cooking for Stroke Patients" is crafted with this in mind, offering practical advice on selecting the right foods, portion control, and meal planning. It simplifies the process of creating meals that are low in sodium, saturated fats, and cholesterol while rich in essential nutrients such as fiber, vitamins, and minerals.

Whether you are a stroke survivor or a caregiver, this book aims to empower you with the knowledge and tools needed to make informed dietary choices. With easy-to-follow instructions, helpful tips, and a variety of recipes that cater to different tastes and preferences, "Healthy Cooking for Stroke Patients" transforms the often-daunting task of dietary change into an enjoyable and fulfilling experience. Embrace the healing power of food and take a proactive step towards recovery and long-term health with this invaluable resource.

Chapter 1

1.1 Understanding Stroke and Recovery

A stroke occurs when the blood supply to part of the brain is interrupted or reduced, preventing brain tissue from getting oxygen and nutrients. This can cause brain cells to begin dying within minutes. There are two main types of strokes:

- **Ischemic Stroke**: Caused by a blockage in an artery that supplies blood to the brain. This is the most common type of stroke.
- **Hemorrhagic Stroke**: Caused by a blood vessel in the brain that bursts, leading to bleeding in or around the brain.

Causes and Risk Factors

Several factors can increase the risk of having a stroke, including:

- **High Blood Pressure**: The leading cause of strokes.
- **Heart Disease**: Conditions such as atrial fibrillation can lead to stroke.
- **Diabetes**: Increases the risk of stroke.

- **Smoking**: Damages blood vessels and raises blood pressure.
- **High Cholesterol**: Can lead to plaque buildup in arteries.
- **Obesity**: Linked to high blood pressure, diabetes, and heart disease.
- **Sedentary Lifestyle**: Lack of physical activity increases risk factors.
- **Excessive Alcohol Consumption**: Raises blood pressure and contributes to obesity.

Symptoms of Stroke

Recognizing stroke symptoms is critical for prompt treatment. Symptoms include:

- Sudden numbness or weakness in the face, arm, or leg, especially on one side of the body.
- Sudden confusion, trouble speaking, or understanding speech.
- Sudden trouble seeing in one or both eyes.
- Sudden trouble walking, dizziness, loss of balance, or lack of coordination.
- Sudden severe headache with no known cause.

The acronym **FAST** is a quick way to remember the symptoms and act fast:

- Face drooping

- Arm weakness
- Speech difficulty
- Time to call emergency services

Stroke Recovery Process

Recovery from a stroke varies depending on the severity and the area of the brain affected. Key aspects of the recovery process include:

- **Medical Treatment**: May involve medication to manage blood pressure, cholesterol, and other conditions.
- **Rehabilitation**: Physical therapy, occupational therapy, and speech therapy are often essential.
- **Lifestyle Changes**: Adopting a healthy diet, increasing physical activity, and quitting smoking are crucial.
- **Support Systems**: Emotional and psychological support from family, friends, and support groups can significantly impact recovery.

Importance of Nutrition in Recovery

Nutrition plays a vital role in the recovery process and long-term health of stroke patients. A well-balanced diet can help:

- **Control Blood Pressure**: Reducing sodium intake and eating a diet rich in fruits, vegetables, and whole grains can lower blood pressure.
- **Manage Cholesterol Levels**: Consuming healthy fats and fiber helps maintain healthy cholesterol levels.
- **Regulate Blood Sugar**: Balanced meals can prevent spikes in blood sugar levels, especially important for those with diabetes.
- **Promote Overall Health**: Adequate nutrition supports the immune system, aids in muscle and tissue repair, and enhances energy levels.

Understanding the intricacies of stroke and the recovery process sets the foundation for implementing dietary and lifestyle changes that can significantly aid in recovery and reduce the risk of future strokes.

1.2 Importance of Nutrition in Stroke Recovery

Nutrition is a critical component in the recovery process for stroke patients. A balanced diet can support healing, improve overall health, and reduce the risk of future strokes. The primary goals of nutrition in stroke recovery include:

- **Reducing Inflammation**: A diet rich in anti-inflammatory foods can help decrease inflammation, which is often elevated after a stroke.
- **Promoting Brain Health**: Certain nutrients are essential for brain function and recovery, such as omega-3 fatty acids, antioxidants, and vitamins.
- **Supporting Cardiovascular Health**: Proper nutrition can help manage blood pressure, cholesterol, and weight, which are all crucial for heart and brain health.

Key Nutrients for Stroke Recovery

1. **Omega-3 Fatty Acids**
   - Found in fish, flaxseeds, and walnuts.
   - Help reduce inflammation and support brain health.

2. **Antioxidants**
   - Present in fruits, vegetables, nuts, and seeds.
   - Protect against oxidative stress and cellular damage.

3. **Vitamins and Minerals**
   - **Vitamin D**: Important for immune function and bone health.

- - **B Vitamins**: Support brain function and energy production.
  - **Magnesium and Potassium**: Help regulate blood pressure and support muscle and nerve function.
4. **Fiber**
   - Found in whole grains, fruits, vegetables, and legumes.
   - Aids in digestive health and helps control blood sugar levels.

Dietary Patterns for Stroke Recovery

1. **DASH Diet (Dietary Approaches to Stop Hypertension)**
   - Emphasizes fruits, vegetables, whole grains, and low-fat dairy.
   - Limits sodium, saturated fat, and added sugars.
   - Proven to lower blood pressure and improve cardiovascular health.

2. **Mediterranean Diet**
   - Focuses on fruits, vegetables, whole grains, nuts, seeds, and olive oil.
   - Includes moderate amounts of fish and poultry, and limits red meat.

- Associated with reduced inflammation and better heart health.

3. **Plant-Based Diet**
   - Centers on vegetables, fruits, whole grains, legumes, nuts, and seeds.
   - Can be tailored to include some animal products if desired.
   - Helps reduce cholesterol levels and supports overall health.

Managing Specific Dietary Needs

1. **Low Sodium Intake**
   - Reducing sodium helps control blood pressure.
   - Aim for less than 2,300 mg of sodium per day, or even lower if advised by a healthcare provider.

2. **Healthy Fats**
   - Choose unsaturated fats like olive oil, avocado, and nuts.
   - Limit saturated fats found in red meat, butter, and full-fat dairy products.
   - Avoid trans fats found in many processed foods.

3. **Blood Sugar Control**
   - Balance carbohydrates with protein and healthy fats.
   - Choose complex carbohydrates like whole grains and legumes.

- Avoid sugary drinks and snacks.

Practical Tips for Implementing a Healthy Diet

1. **Meal Planning**
   - Plan meals and snacks in advance to ensure a balanced diet.
   - Include a variety of foods to meet nutritional needs.
2. **Cooking Methods**
   - Use healthier cooking methods like grilling, baking, steaming, and sautéing.
   - Avoid deep-frying and excessive use of oil and butter.
3. **Portion Control**
   - Be mindful of portion sizes to maintain a healthy weight.
   - Use smaller plates and bowls to help control portions.
4. **Reading Nutrition Labels**
   - Check labels for sodium, added sugars, and unhealthy fats.
   - Choose products with higher fiber and nutrient content.

The Role of Hydration

1. **Importance of Staying Hydrated**

- Adequate hydration supports overall health and recovery.
- Dehydration can lead to complications and hinder recovery.

2. **Hydration Tips**
   - Drink plenty of water throughout the day.
   - Limit caffeinated and sugary beverages.
   - Include hydrating foods like fruits and vegetables in the diet.

Proper nutrition is vital for stroke recovery, playing a crucial role in healing, reducing the risk of recurrent strokes, and promoting overall health and well-being.

Chapter 2

2.1 Essential Nutrients for Stroke Recovery

Proper nutrition is crucial for stroke recovery as it supports healing, boosts energy, and helps prevent future strokes. Here are some essential nutrients that play a significant role in this process:

Omega-3 Fatty Acids

- **Sources**: Fatty fish (salmon, mackerel, sardines), flaxseeds, chia seeds, walnuts, and fish oil supplements.
- **Benefits**: Omega-3 fatty acids reduce inflammation, support brain health, improve cognitive function, and promote cardiovascular health.

Antioxidants

- **Sources**: Berries (blueberries, strawberries), dark leafy greens (spinach, kale), nuts (almonds, walnuts), seeds, dark chocolate, and green tea.
- **Benefits**: Antioxidants help protect brain cells from oxidative stress and damage,

which is crucial for recovery and overall brain function.

Vitamins

1. **Vitamin D**
   - ○ **Sources**: Sunlight exposure, fatty fish, fortified dairy products, and supplements.
   - ○ **Benefits**: Supports immune function, bone health, and may play a role in brain health.
2. **B Vitamins (B6, B12, Folate)**
   - ○ **Sources**: Whole grains, leafy greens, legumes, nuts, seeds, eggs, dairy products, and meat.
   - ○ **Benefits**: Important for energy production, nerve function, and reducing homocysteine levels, which is linked to a lower risk of stroke.
3. **Vitamin C**
   - ○ **Sources**: Citrus fruits (oranges, lemons), strawberries, bell peppers, broccoli, and Brussels sprouts.
   - ○ **Benefits**: Enhances immune function and acts as an antioxidant to protect brain cells.
4. **Vitamin E**
   - ○ **Sources**: Nuts, seeds, spinach, broccoli, and vegetable oils.

- ○ **Benefits**: Protects cells from oxidative damage and supports brain health.

Minerals

1. **Magnesium**
   - ○ **Sources**: Leafy greens, nuts, seeds, whole grains, and legumes.
   - ○ **Benefits**: Helps regulate blood pressure, supports nerve function, and reduces the risk of stroke.
2. **Potassium**
   - ○ **Sources**: Bananas, oranges, potatoes, tomatoes, spinach, and beans.
   - ○ **Benefits**: Helps maintain normal blood pressure and supports heart health.
3. **Calcium**
   - ○ **Sources**: Dairy products, leafy greens, fortified plant-based milk, and tofu.
   - ○ **Benefits**: Essential for bone health and may help regulate blood pressure.

Protein

- **Sources**: Lean meats (chicken, turkey), fish, eggs, dairy products, legumes, nuts, seeds, and soy products.
- **Benefits**: Essential for tissue repair, muscle maintenance, and overall recovery.

Fiber

- **Sources**: Whole grains, fruits, vegetables, legumes, nuts, and seeds.
- **Benefits**: Aids in digestive health, helps control blood sugar levels, and lowers cholesterol levels.

Healthy Fats

- **Sources**: Avocados, olive oil, nuts, seeds, and fatty fish.
- **Benefits**: Supports brain health, reduces inflammation, and promotes heart health.

Water

- **Sources**: Drinking water, herbal teas, and water-rich foods like fruits and vegetables.
- **Benefits**: Maintains hydration, aids in digestion, and supports overall bodily functions.

Phytochemicals

- **Sources**: Fruits, vegetables, whole grains, nuts, seeds, and legumes.
- **Benefits**: These plant compounds have various health benefits, including anti-

inflammatory and antioxidant properties that support recovery and overall health.

Ensuring that a stroke patient's diet includes these essential nutrients can significantly enhance their recovery process, promote brain and heart health, and reduce the risk of future strokes.

2.2 Role of Vitamins and Minerals

Vitamins and minerals play a vital role in the recovery process for stroke patients. They support various bodily functions, enhance overall health, and aid in healing. Here is an overview of key vitamins and minerals essential for stroke recovery:

Vitamins

1. **Vitamin D**
    - **Sources**: Sunlight exposure, fatty fish (salmon, mackerel), fortified dairy products, and supplements.
    - **Benefits**: Enhances immune function, supports bone health, and may contribute to brain health. Adequate levels of vitamin D are associated with reduced inflammation and improved mood.
2. **B Vitamins**

- ○ **Sources**: Whole grains, leafy greens, legumes, nuts, seeds, eggs, dairy products, meat, and fish.
- ○ **Benefits**:
    - ■ **Vitamin B6 (Pyridoxine)**: Supports brain health and neurotransmitter function.
    - ■ **Vitamin B12 (Cobalamin)**: Essential for nerve function and the production of red blood cells. Helps maintain cognitive function and reduces the risk of memory loss.
    - ■ **Folate (Vitamin B9)**: Important for DNA synthesis and repair. Reduces homocysteine levels, which are linked to a higher risk of cardiovascular diseases and stroke.

3. **Vitamin C**
- ○ **Sources**: Citrus fruits (oranges, lemons), strawberries, bell peppers, broccoli, Brussels sprouts, and tomatoes.
- ○ **Benefits**: Acts as an antioxidant to protect brain cells from damage, enhances immune function, and supports the healing of tissues.

4. **Vitamin E**

- **Sources**: Nuts, seeds, spinach, broccoli, and vegetable oils.
    - **Benefits**: Antioxidant properties protect cells from oxidative stress and damage. Supports brain health and reduces inflammation.
5. **Vitamin K**
    - **Sources**: Leafy greens (kale, spinach, broccoli), Brussels sprouts, and green beans.
    - **Benefits**: Important for blood clotting and bone health. Helps regulate calcium in the blood and bones.

Minerals

1. **Magnesium**
    - **Sources**: Leafy greens, nuts, seeds, whole grains, and legumes.
    - **Benefits**: Helps regulate blood pressure, supports nerve and muscle function, and contributes to heart health. Magnesium deficiency is linked to an increased risk of stroke.
2. **Potassium**
    - **Sources**: Bananas, oranges, potatoes, tomatoes, spinach, beans, and avocados.
    - **Benefits**: Helps maintain normal blood pressure, supports heart

function, and regulates fluid balance. Adequate potassium intake can reduce the risk of stroke.

3. **Calcium**
   - **Sources**: Dairy products, leafy greens, fortified plant-based milk, tofu, and almonds.
   - **Benefits**: Essential for bone health and muscle function. May help regulate blood pressure when combined with other nutrients like magnesium and potassium.

4. **Zinc**
   - **Sources**: Meat, shellfish, legumes, seeds, nuts, dairy products, and whole grains.
   - **Benefits**: Supports immune function, aids in wound healing, and is important for brain function. Zinc deficiency can impair cognitive function and recovery.

5. **Iron**
   - **Sources**: Red meat, poultry, fish, legumes, fortified cereals, and spinach.
   - **Benefits**: Essential for the production of hemoglobin, which carries oxygen in the blood. Adequate iron levels prevent anemia, which can cause fatigue and hinder recovery.

6. **Selenium**

- ○ **Sources**: Brazil nuts, seafood, meats, and whole grains.
- ○ **Benefits**: Acts as an antioxidant, supports immune function, and protects against oxidative damage.

Integrating Vitamins and Minerals into the Diet

1. **Balanced Diet**
   - ○ Incorporate a variety of foods to ensure a comprehensive intake of vitamins and minerals.
   - ○ Focus on whole foods like fruits, vegetables, whole grains, lean proteins, nuts, and seeds.
2. **Supplements**
   - ○ Consider supplements if dietary intake is insufficient, but consult with a healthcare provider before starting any new supplement regimen.

3. **Cooking Methods**
   - ○ Use cooking methods that preserve nutrients, such as steaming, grilling, and baking.
   - ○ Avoid overcooking, which can deplete vitamins and minerals.

Ensuring an adequate intake of essential vitamins and minerals through a balanced diet or supplements can significantly enhance the recovery process for stroke patients, supporting overall health and well-being.

2.3 Hydration Needs

Proper hydration is crucial for stroke recovery. Dehydration can hinder the healing process and exacerbate symptoms. Here's an overview of the hydration needs for stroke patients:

Importance of Hydration

1. **Brain Function**
   - Water is essential for brain function. Proper hydration supports cognitive processes, memory, and overall brain health.
2. **Circulation**
   - Adequate fluid intake ensures proper blood circulation, which is vital for delivering oxygen and nutrients to the brain and other tissues.
3. **Detoxification**

- Hydration helps flush out toxins from the body, which can be beneficial for overall health and recovery.

4. **Temperature Regulation**
   - Water helps regulate body temperature, which is important for maintaining homeostasis, especially during physical activity.

5. **Digestive Health**
   - Proper hydration aids in digestion and prevents constipation, which is a common issue for stroke patients due to reduced mobility and medication side effects.

Hydration Guidelines

1. **General Recommendations**
   - Aim for at least 8-10 cups (2-2.5 liters) of fluids per day. This can vary based on individual needs, activity levels, and climate.

2. **Individual Needs**
   - Consider factors like body weight, physical activity, and medical conditions when determining fluid needs. Consulting with a healthcare provider can help tailor specific recommendations.

Sources of Hydration

1. **Water**
   - The best source of hydration. Aim to drink water throughout the day rather than consuming large amounts at once.
2. **Herbal Teas**
   - Caffeine-free herbal teas are a good alternative to water and can provide additional health benefits.
3. **Infused Water**
   - Adding slices of fruits, vegetables, or herbs to water can make it more appealing and add nutrients.
4. **Broths and Soups**
   - These can contribute to daily fluid intake and provide essential nutrients, especially if made with nutrient-rich ingredients.
5. **Hydrating Foods**
   - Many fruits and vegetables have high water content. Examples include cucumbers, watermelon, oranges, and strawberries.

Signs of Dehydration

1. **Early Signs**
   - Thirst, dry mouth, dark yellow urine, and reduced urine output.

2. **Severe Signs**
    - Dizziness, confusion, rapid heartbeat, and fainting. These require immediate medical attention.

Strategies to Ensure Adequate Hydration

1. **Regular Drinking Schedule**
    - Establish a routine to drink fluids at regular intervals throughout the day, even if not feeling thirsty.
2. **Use of Reminders**
    - Use alarms or smartphone apps to remind the patient to drink water.
3. **Easily Accessible Fluids**
    - Keep water bottles or glasses of water within easy reach, especially for those with mobility issues.
4. **Monitoring Fluid Intake**
    - Keep a log or use a tracking app to monitor daily fluid intake and ensure goals are being met.
5. **Adjusting Fluid Intake**
    - Increase fluid intake during hot weather, physical activity, or illness to compensate for additional fluid loss.

Proper hydration is essential for supporting brain function, circulation, detoxification, temperature regulation, and digestive health in stroke patients.

Ensuring adequate fluid intake through various sources and strategies can significantly enhance the recovery process.

Chapter 3

3.1 Low Sodium Diet

A low sodium diet is crucial for stroke patients as it helps manage blood pressure, reduce the risk of recurrent strokes, and improve overall cardiovascular health. Here's a detailed guide on implementing a low sodium diet:

Importance of Reducing Sodium

1. **Blood Pressure Control**
   - High sodium intake is linked to increased blood pressure, a significant risk factor for strokes.
2. **Heart Health**
   - Lowering sodium can reduce the strain on the cardiovascular system and improve heart health.
3. **Fluid Balance**
   - Reducing sodium intake helps maintain proper fluid balance and prevent fluid retention, which can strain the heart and blood vessels.

Recommended Sodium Intake

1. **General Guidelines**

- The American Heart Association recommends no more than 2,300 milligrams (mg) of sodium per day, with an ideal limit of 1,500 mg for most adults, especially those with high blood pressure or a history of stroke.

2. **Individual Needs**
   - Specific recommendations may vary based on individual health conditions. Consult a healthcare provider for personalized advice.

Identifying High Sodium Foods

1. **Processed Foods**
   - Canned soups, processed meats (bacon, ham, sausages), frozen meals, and snack foods (chips, crackers) are typically high in sodium.
2. **Restaurant and Fast Foods**
   - Many restaurant and fast food items contain high levels of sodium due to added salt and preservatives.
3. **Condiments and Sauces**
   - Soy sauce, ketchup, salad dressings, and seasoning mixes can contribute significant amounts of sodium.
4. **Packaged Snacks**
   - Pretzels, salted nuts, and popcorn often have high sodium content.

Strategies for Reducing Sodium Intake

1. **Cooking at Home**
    - Preparing meals at home allows for better control over sodium content. Use fresh ingredients and minimize the use of salt.
2. **Reading Nutrition Labels**
    - Check labels for sodium content and choose products with lower sodium levels. Aim for items with less than 140 mg of sodium per serving.
3. **Using Herbs and Spices**
    - Enhance flavor with herbs, spices, garlic, lemon juice, and vinegar instead of salt.
4. **Choosing Fresh or Frozen Vegetables**
    - Opt for fresh or frozen vegetables without added sauces or seasonings.
5. **Rinsing Canned Foods**
    - Rinse canned beans, vegetables, and fish to remove excess sodium.
6. **Low-Sodium Alternatives**
    - Select low-sodium or no-salt-added versions of foods like broth, soy sauce, and snacks.
7. **Portion Control**
    - Be mindful of portion sizes to help manage overall sodium intake.

Sample Low Sodium Meal Plan

1. **Breakfast**
    - **Oatmeal** with fresh berries and a sprinkle of cinnamon.
    - **Smoothie** with spinach, banana, and almond milk.
2. **Lunch**
    - **Grilled Chicken Salad** with mixed greens, cherry tomatoes, cucumbers, and a homemade vinaigrette (olive oil, vinegar, and herbs).
    - **Vegetable Soup** made with low-sodium broth and a variety of fresh vegetables.
3. **Dinner**
    - **Baked Salmon** with a squeeze of lemon and a side of steamed broccoli and quinoa.
    - **Stuffed Bell Peppers** with a filling of brown rice, black beans, corn, and diced tomatoes (no salt added).
4. **Snacks**
    - **Fresh Fruit** (apple, orange, or banana).
    - **Unsalted Nuts** or **Plain Yogurt** with a drizzle of honey.

Monitoring Progress

1. **Track Sodium Intake**
   - Use a food diary or an app to track daily sodium consumption and stay within recommended limits.
2. **Regular Health Checkups**
   - Monitor blood pressure and overall health with regular visits to a healthcare provider to ensure the diet is effective.
3. **Adjustments as Needed**
   - Make dietary adjustments based on feedback from health professionals and any observed changes in health status.

A low sodium diet is a key component of stroke recovery, helping to control blood pressure and support heart health. By making informed food choices and incorporating healthy habits, stroke patients can significantly improve their overall well-being.

3.2 Managing Cholesterol and Fat Intake

Controlling cholesterol and fat intake is vital for stroke recovery and prevention. A diet low in unhealthy fats and cholesterol can help manage cardiovascular health and reduce the risk of recurrent strokes. Here's how to manage cholesterol and fat intake effectively:

Understanding Cholesterol and Fat

1. **Cholesterol**
   - **Types:**
     - **LDL (Low-Density Lipoprotein)**: Known as "bad" cholesterol, high levels can lead to plaque buildup in arteries.
     - **HDL (High-Density Lipoprotein)**: Known as "good" cholesterol, helps remove LDL cholesterol from the bloodstream.
   - **Sources**: Found in animal products like meat, dairy, and eggs.
2. **Fat**
   - **Types:**
     - **Saturated Fats**: Found in animal products and some plant

oils. Can raise LDL cholesterol levels.
- **Trans Fats**: Found in many processed foods. Raises LDL and lowers HDL cholesterol, increasing heart disease risk.
- **Unsaturated Fats**: Includes monounsaturated and polyunsaturated fats found in plant oils, nuts, seeds, and fish. Beneficial for heart health.

Recommended Intake

1. **Cholesterol**
   - Limit dietary cholesterol to less than 300 mg per day. For those with heart disease or stroke history, aim for less than 200 mg per day.
2. **Fat**
   - **Total Fat**: Should comprise 25-35% of daily calories.
   - **Saturated Fat**: Limit to less than 7% of daily calories.
   - **Trans Fat**: Avoid as much as possible.
   - **Unsaturated Fat**: Focus on sources of healthy fats, making up the remainder of the daily fat intake.

Dietary Strategies to Manage Cholesterol and Fat

1. **Choosing Healthy Fats**
   - **Sources of Unsaturated Fats**: Olive oil, canola oil, avocados, nuts, seeds, and fatty fish (salmon, mackerel, sardines).
   - **Avoiding Trans Fats**: Steer clear of partially hydrogenated oils found in many fried and baked goods.
2. **Reducing Saturated Fats**
   - **Lean Meats**: Choose lean cuts of meat, poultry without skin, and fish.
   - **Dairy Products**: Opt for low-fat or fat-free dairy products.
   - **Cooking Methods**: Grill, bake, steam, or sauté instead of frying.
3. **Increasing Fiber Intake**
   - **Soluble Fiber**: Found in oats, beans, lentils, fruits, and vegetables. Helps lower LDL cholesterol.
   - **Whole Grains**: Replace refined grains with whole grains like brown rice, quinoa, and whole wheat.
4. **Incorporating Plant-Based Foods**
   - **Legumes and Nuts**: Beans, lentils, chickpeas, almonds, and walnuts are excellent sources of protein and healthy fats.

- Fruits and Vegetables: Aim for a variety of colorful fruits and vegetables to ensure a range of nutrients and antioxidants.

5. **Reading Nutrition Labels**
   - **Checking Fat Content**: Look for foods with low saturated and trans fat content.
   - **Watching Cholesterol Levels**: Select products with lower cholesterol amounts.
6. **Reducing Red Meat Consumption**
   - **Plant-Based Proteins**: Incorporate more plant-based proteins like beans, tofu, and tempeh.
   - **Fish and Poultry**: Increase consumption of fish and poultry as alternatives to red meat.

Sample Meal Plan for Managing Cholesterol and Fat

1. **Breakfast**
   - **Oatmeal** with berries, chia seeds, and a splash of almond milk.
   - **Smoothie** with spinach, banana, flaxseeds, and low-fat yogurt.
2. **Lunch**

- o **Quinoa Salad** with mixed greens, cherry tomatoes, cucumber, avocado, and a lemon-tahini dressing.
    - o **Lentil Soup** made with a variety of vegetables and herbs.
3. **Dinner**
    - o **Baked Salmon** with a side of roasted Brussels sprouts and sweet potato.
    - o **Stir-Fried Tofu** with broccoli, bell peppers, and brown rice.
4. **Snacks**
    - o **Fresh Fruit**: Apple slices with a small handful of walnuts.
    - o **Vegetable Sticks**: Carrot and celery sticks with hummus.

Monitoring Progress

1. **Regular Checkups**
    - o Have regular blood tests to monitor cholesterol levels and adjust the diet as necessary.
2. **Lifestyle Adjustments**
    - o Combine dietary changes with regular physical activity, smoking cessation, and stress management for optimal heart health.
3. **Dietary Tracking**

- ○ Use food diaries or apps to track fat
    and cholesterol intake, helping stay
    within recommended limits.

Managing cholesterol and fat intake through a balanced diet rich in healthy fats, fiber, and plant-based foods is essential for stroke recovery and cardiovascular health. Implementing these strategies can significantly reduce the risk of future strokes and improve overall well-being.

3.3 Controlling Blood Sugar Levels

Managing blood sugar levels is crucial for stroke recovery, particularly for patients with diabetes or those at risk of developing diabetes. High blood sugar can damage blood vessels and nerves, increasing the risk of recurrent strokes and other complications. Here's a detailed guide on controlling blood sugar levels:

Understanding Blood Sugar and Stroke Risk

1. **Connection Between Diabetes and Stroke**
   - ○ Diabetes increases the risk of stroke
     due to its impact on blood vessels and

the likelihood of developing high
blood pressure and high cholesterol.

2. **Impact of High Blood Sugar**
    - Elevated blood sugar levels can cause
      inflammation and damage to blood
      vessels, contributing to the formation
      of blood clots and plaque buildup in
      arteries.

Recommended Blood Sugar Levels

1. **Fasting Blood Sugar**
    - Aim for 70-130 mg/dL before meals.
2. **Postprandial (After Meals) Blood Sugar**
    - Target less than 180 mg/dL one to two
      hours after eating.
3. **Hemoglobin A1c**
    - Aim for an HbA1c level below 7% for
      most adults with diabetes. Individual
      targets may vary based on personal
      health conditions.

Dietary Strategies for Blood Sugar Control

1. **Balanced Meals**
    - Combine carbohydrates with protein
      and healthy fats to slow digestion and
      prevent blood sugar spikes.
2. **Choosing Low Glycemic Index (GI) Foods**

- Opt for low GI foods that have a slower, more gradual impact on blood sugar levels. Examples include whole grains, legumes, vegetables, and most fruits.

3. **Portion Control**
   - Monitor portion sizes to avoid consuming too many carbohydrates at once. Use measuring tools or visual aids to keep portions in check.

4. **Regular Meal Timing**
   - Eat at consistent times throughout the day to maintain stable blood sugar levels. Avoid skipping meals, which can lead to overeating and blood sugar fluctuations.

5. **Healthy Snacks**
   - Choose snacks that combine protein and fiber, such as apple slices with peanut butter or a handful of nuts and seeds.

6. **Limiting Sugary Foods and Drinks**
   - Avoid sugary beverages (soda, fruit juices) and limit sweets and desserts. Choose water, unsweetened tea, or coffee instead.

Nutrient-Rich Foods for Blood Sugar Control

1. **Fiber-Rich Foods**

- Whole grains (oats, barley, quinoa), legumes (beans, lentils), fruits, and vegetables.
- **Benefits**: Fiber slows carbohydrate absorption, helping to maintain stable blood sugar levels.

2. **Healthy Fats**
   - Sources include avocados, nuts, seeds, olive oil, and fatty fish (salmon, mackerel).
   - **Benefits**: Healthy fats improve satiety and support overall cardiovascular health.

3. **Lean Proteins**
   - Choose lean meats (chicken, turkey), fish, eggs, tofu, and low-fat dairy products.
   - **Benefits**: Protein helps control hunger and maintain muscle mass, which is essential for recovery.

4. **Non-Starchy Vegetables**
   - Include a variety of vegetables like spinach, broccoli, bell peppers, and cauliflower.
   - **Benefits**: Low in calories and carbohydrates, high in essential nutrients and fiber.

Sample Meal Plan for Blood Sugar Control

1. **Breakfast**
    - **Vegetable Omelette**: Made with spinach, tomatoes, and mushrooms.
    - **Whole Grain Toast**: One slice with a thin spread of avocado.
2. **Lunch**
    - **Grilled Chicken Salad**: Mixed greens, cucumbers, cherry tomatoes, and a small amount of olive oil and vinegar.
    - **Quinoa**: Half a cup as a side dish.
3. **Dinner**
    - **Baked Fish**: Seasoned with herbs and a squeeze of lemon.
    - **Steamed Vegetables**: Broccoli, carrots, and zucchini.
    - **Brown Rice**: One serving (about 1/2 cup).
4. **Snacks**
    - **Greek Yogurt**: Plain, with a handful of berries.
    - **Mixed Nuts**: A small handful (about 1 ounce).

Monitoring and Managing Blood Sugar Levels

1. **Regular Monitoring**
    - Use a blood glucose monitor to check levels regularly. Keep a log to track patterns and identify any fluctuations.

2. **Physical Activity**
   - Incorporate regular exercise, such as walking, swimming, or yoga. Physical activity helps lower blood sugar levels and improve insulin sensitivity.
3. **Medication Adherence**
   - Follow prescribed medications and insulin regimens as directed by healthcare providers.
4. **Stress Management**
   - Practice stress-reducing techniques like deep breathing, meditation, and mindfulness. Stress can impact blood sugar levels.
5. **Healthcare Support**
   - Work with healthcare providers to adjust treatment plans as needed. Regular check-ups are essential for managing diabetes and reducing stroke risk.

Controlling blood sugar levels through a balanced diet, regular monitoring, and healthy lifestyle choices is vital for stroke recovery and preventing future complications. Implementing these strategies can support overall health and improve outcomes for stroke patients.

3.4 Increasing Fiber Intake

Fiber plays a crucial role in overall health, particularly in managing cholesterol levels, blood sugar levels, and promoting digestive health. For stroke patients, increasing fiber intake can aid in recovery and reduce the risk of recurrent strokes. Here's how to effectively increase fiber intake:

Benefits of Fiber for Stroke Recovery

1. **Heart Health**
   - Soluble fiber helps lower LDL cholesterol, reducing the risk of cardiovascular diseases and subsequent strokes.
2. **Blood Sugar Control**
   - Fiber slows the absorption of sugar, helping to maintain stable blood sugar levels, which is especially beneficial for stroke patients with diabetes.
3. **Digestive Health**
   - Fiber aids in regular bowel movements and prevents constipation, a common issue for stroke patients due to reduced mobility and medication side effects.
4. **Weight Management**

- High-fiber foods are more filling, which can help manage weight, an important factor in reducing stroke risk.

Recommended Fiber Intake

1. **General Guidelines**
   - The recommended daily intake of fiber is 25 grams for women and 38 grams for men. For those over 50, the recommendation is 21 grams for women and 30 grams for men.
2. **Gradual Increase**
   - Increase fiber intake gradually to prevent digestive discomfort such as bloating and gas. Aim to add a few grams of fiber per week until reaching the recommended levels.

High-Fiber Foods to Include

1. **Fruits**
   - Apples, pears, berries (strawberries, raspberries, blueberries), bananas, and oranges.

2. **Vegetables**

- Broccoli, carrots, spinach, kale, Brussels sprouts, and sweet potatoes.

3. **Whole Grains**
   - Oats, brown rice, quinoa, barley, whole wheat bread, and whole grain cereals.
4. **Legumes**
   - Beans (black beans, kidney beans, chickpeas), lentils, and peas.
5. **Nuts and Seeds**
   - Almonds, chia seeds, flaxseeds, and sunflower seeds.

Strategies to Increase Fiber Intake

1. **Incorporate Fiber-Rich Foods in Every Meal**
   - **Breakfast**: Add berries or sliced fruit to oatmeal or yogurt. Choose whole grain cereals.
   - **Lunch**: Include a side salad with mixed greens, vegetables, and legumes. Use whole grain bread for sandwiches.
   - **Dinner**: Opt for whole grains like brown rice or quinoa. Add extra vegetables to soups, stews, and casseroles.

- ○ **Snacks**: Choose raw vegetables with hummus, fresh fruit, or a handful of nuts.
2. **Replace Refined Grains with Whole Grains**
   - ○ Swap white bread, rice, and pasta for their whole grain counterparts.
3. **Add Legumes to Meals**
   - ○ Incorporate beans or lentils into soups, stews, salads, and side dishes.
4. **Snack on High-Fiber Foods**
   - ○ Keep high-fiber snacks like fruit, nuts, and whole grain crackers readily available.
5. **Experiment with Fiber Supplements**
   - ○ If dietary changes are not enough, consider fiber supplements such as psyllium husk. Consult with a healthcare provider before starting any supplements.

Sample High-Fiber Meal Plan

1. **Breakfast**
   - ○ **Oatmeal** with sliced bananas and a sprinkle of chia seeds.
   - ○ **Smoothie**: Spinach, berries, flaxseeds, and almond milk.

2. **Lunch**
    - o **Quinoa Salad**: Mixed greens, cherry tomatoes, cucumber, chickpeas, and a lemon-tahini dressing.
    - o **Lentil Soup**: Made with a variety of vegetables and herbs.
3. **Dinner**
    - o **Grilled Salmon** with a side of steamed broccoli and sweet potato.
    - o **Vegetable Stir-Fry**: Bell peppers, broccoli, carrots, and tofu over brown rice.
4. **Snacks**
    - o **Apple Slices** with almond butter.
    - o **Carrot and Celery Sticks** with hummus.
    - o **Mixed Nuts**: A small handful (about 1 ounce).

Tips for Successful Fiber Integration

1. **Hydration**
    - o Drink plenty of water when increasing fiber intake to help fiber move through the digestive system and prevent constipation.
2. **Cooking Methods**
    - o Use cooking methods that retain fiber content, such as steaming, baking, and roasting.

3. **Reading Labels**
    - Check nutrition labels for fiber content and choose products with higher fiber amounts.
4. **Consistency**
    - Make fiber intake a regular part of the diet rather than sporadic. Consistency is key for reaping the benefits of fiber.

Increasing fiber intake through a balanced diet rich in fruits, vegetables, whole grains, legumes, nuts, and seeds can significantly enhance stroke recovery. Implementing these strategies will support cardiovascular health, blood sugar control, and overall well-being.

Chapter 4

4.1 Creating Balanced Meal Plans

Balanced meal plans are essential for stroke recovery, ensuring that patients receive the right nutrients to support healing and overall health. A well-rounded diet can help manage blood pressure, cholesterol, blood sugar levels, and provide the energy needed for rehabilitation. Here's how to create balanced meal plans:

Key Components of a Balanced Meal Plan

1. **Macronutrients**
   - **Carbohydrates**: Focus on complex carbs like whole grains, fruits, and vegetables.
   - **Proteins**: Include lean meats, fish, legumes, dairy, and plant-based proteins.
   - **Fats**: Opt for healthy fats from avocados, nuts, seeds, and olive oil.
2. **Micronutrients**
   - **Vitamins and Minerals**: Ensure a variety of fruits and vegetables to provide essential vitamins and minerals such as potassium, magnesium, and vitamins A, C, and K.
3. **Fiber**
   - Integrate high-fiber foods to support digestive health, control blood sugar, and lower cholesterol.
4. **Hydration**
   - Include adequate fluids, primarily water, to stay hydrated and support bodily functions.

Meal Planning Guidelines

1. **Variety**
   - Incorporate a wide range of foods to cover all nutrient needs and prevent meal fatigue.

2. **Portion Control**
    - Use appropriate portion sizes to avoid overeating and manage weight.
3. **Balanced Macronutrients**
    - Ensure each meal contains a good balance of carbs, protein, and healthy fats.

4. **Consistent Meal Times**
    - Plan meals and snacks at regular intervals to maintain stable energy levels and blood sugar.

Sample 7-Day Balanced Meal Plan

Day 1

- **Breakfast**: Greek yogurt with mixed berries and a sprinkle of chia seeds.
- **Lunch**: Quinoa salad with black beans, corn, cherry tomatoes, avocado, and lime dressing.
- **Dinner**: Grilled chicken breast with steamed broccoli and brown rice.
- **Snack**: Apple slices with almond butter.

Day 2

- **Breakfast**: Oatmeal topped with sliced banana and walnuts.

- **Lunch**: Lentil soup with a side of mixed greens salad.
- **Dinner**: Baked salmon with roasted Brussels sprouts and sweet potato.
- **Snack**: Carrot and celery sticks with hummus.

Day 3

- **Breakfast**: Whole grain toast with avocado and a poached egg.
- **Lunch**: Turkey and vegetable wrap with whole grain tortilla.
- **Dinner**: Stir-fried tofu with bell peppers, snap peas, and brown rice.
- **Snack**: Greek yogurt with a handful of nuts.

Day 4

- **Breakfast**: Smoothie with spinach, frozen berries, banana, and flaxseed.
- **Lunch**: Chickpea and vegetable stew with whole grain bread.
- **Dinner**: Grilled shrimp with quinoa and steamed asparagus.
- **Snack**: Fresh fruit salad.

Day 5

- **Breakfast**: Cottage cheese with pineapple and a sprinkle of cinnamon.

- **Lunch**: Chicken and vegetable stir-fry with brown rice.
- **Dinner**: Baked cod with a side of mixed vegetables and whole wheat couscous.
- **Snack**: Handful of mixed nuts.

Day 6

- **Breakfast**: Whole grain cereal with almond milk and sliced strawberries.
- **Lunch**: Black bean and avocado salad with lime dressing.
- **Dinner**: Turkey meatloaf with mashed cauliflower and green beans.
- **Snack**: Sliced bell peppers with guacamole.

Day 7

- **Breakfast**: Scrambled eggs with spinach, tomatoes, and whole grain toast.
- **Lunch**: Tuna salad with mixed greens, cucumbers, and olive oil dressing.
- **Dinner**: Vegetable and lentil curry with brown rice.
- **Snack**: Smoothie with kale, apple, and ginger.

Tips for Meal Preparation

1. **Plan Ahead**
   - Create a weekly meal plan and shopping list to ensure all necessary ingredients are available.
2. **Batch Cooking**
   - Prepare larger quantities of meals and portion them out for the week to save time and ensure consistency.
3. **Incorporate Leftovers**
   - Use leftovers creatively to prevent waste and reduce cooking time.
4. **Use Healthy Cooking Methods**
   - Opt for grilling, baking, steaming, and sautéing with minimal oil.
5. **Portion Control**
   - Use measuring cups, a food scale, or visual cues to maintain appropriate portion sizes.
6. **Stay Hydrated**
   - Include water, herbal teas, and other low-calorie beverages throughout the day.
7. **Monitor Nutrient Intake**
   - Use a food diary or app to track nutrient intake and ensure a balanced diet.

Creating balanced meal plans involves incorporating a variety of nutrient-dense foods, maintaining portion control, and ensuring regular meals and snacks. This approach supports stroke recovery by providing essential nutrients, managing blood sugar, cholesterol, and promoting overall health.

4.2 Tips for Easy Meal Preparation

Meal preparation can be streamlined to ensure that stroke patients get the necessary nutrients without spending excessive time and effort in the kitchen. Here are practical tips for easy meal preparation:

Planning and Organization

1. **Create a Weekly Meal Plan**
   - Outline meals for the week, considering breakfast, lunch, dinner, and snacks. This reduces daily decision-making and ensures balanced nutrition.

2. **Make a Shopping List**
   - Based on the meal plan, create a detailed shopping list to ensure all necessary ingredients are available.

3. **Organize the Kitchen**
   - Keep commonly used items, such as cooking utensils, spices, and pantry staples, easily accessible to save time during cooking.

Efficient Cooking Strategies

1. **Batch Cooking**
   - Prepare larger quantities of meals that can be stored and reheated throughout the week. This reduces daily cooking time and ensures ready-to-eat meals.
2. **One-Pot Meals**
   - Utilize recipes that can be made in a single pot or pan, such as soups, stews, and casseroles, to minimize cleanup and cooking time.
3. **Sheet Pan Meals**
   - Cook entire meals on a single baking sheet, combining proteins and vegetables for easy preparation and cleanup.
4. **Slow Cooker and Instant Pot**
   - Use slow cookers or Instant Pots to prepare meals with minimal hands-on time. These appliances are excellent for soups, stews, and braised dishes.

Smart Ingredient Choices

1. **Pre-Cut Vegetables**
   - Purchase pre-cut or frozen vegetables to save time on chopping and cleaning.
2. **Canned and Frozen Foods**
   - Use canned beans, tomatoes, and frozen fruits and vegetables. They are convenient and retain most of their nutritional value.
3. **Lean Proteins**
   - Opt for quick-cooking proteins like chicken breasts, fish fillets, and plant-based options like tofu or tempeh.

Time-Saving Techniques

1. **Prep Ingredients in Advance**
   - Wash, chop, and portion out ingredients ahead of time, storing them in containers for quick assembly during the week.
2. **Use Kitchen Gadgets**
   - Utilize tools like food processors, blenders, and mandolins to speed up food preparation tasks.
3. **Cook Once, Eat Twice**
   - Double recipes and freeze half for future meals, reducing the need to cook every day.
4. **Simplify Recipes**

- Choose recipes with fewer ingredients and straightforward steps to minimize preparation time.

Easy and Nutritious Meal Ideas

1. **Breakfast**
   - **Overnight Oats**: Combine oats, milk (or plant-based alternative), and your choice of fruit and nuts in a jar. Refrigerate overnight.
   - **Smoothies**: Blend fruits, vegetables, protein powder, and liquid for a quick and nutritious meal.
2. **Lunch**
   - **Salads in a Jar**: Layer ingredients (dressing at the bottom, followed by vegetables and protein) in a jar for a portable, ready-to-eat meal.
   - **Wraps**: Use whole grain tortillas to wrap lean protein, vegetables, and a healthy spread like hummus or avocado.
3. **Dinner**
   - **Stir-Fries**: Quickly cook vegetables and protein in a single pan with a simple sauce. Serve over brown rice or quinoa.
   - **Sheet Pan Dinners**: Roast a combination of protein and vegetables

on a baking sheet with olive oil and spices.

4. **Snacks**
    - **Fruit and Nut Mixes**: Combine dried fruits and nuts for a quick, portable snack.
    - **Vegetable Sticks and Hummus**: Pre-cut vegetables like carrots, celery, and bell peppers served with hummus.

Practical Tips

1. **Stay Organized**
    - Keep a clean and organized kitchen workspace to streamline cooking and cleanup.
2. **Label and Date Food**
    - Use labels and dates on containers to keep track of prepared meals and ingredients, ensuring freshness and reducing waste.
3. **Use Leftovers Wisely**
    - Repurpose leftovers into new meals, such as turning roasted vegetables into a soup or using cooked chicken in a salad.
4. **Involve Family Members**
    - Share meal prep tasks with family members or caregivers to distribute the

workload and make the process more enjoyable.

5. **Keep it Simple**
   - Focus on simple, nutritious meals that are easy to prepare and require minimal ingredients.

By incorporating these tips into the meal preparation routine, stroke patients can enjoy nutritious, balanced meals with less effort and time, supporting their recovery and overall health.

4.3 Batch Cooking and Freezing

Batch cooking and freezing meals can be a game-changer for stroke patients and their caregivers, offering convenience, time savings, and consistent access to nutritious meals. Here's a guide on how to effectively batch cook and freeze meals:

Benefits of Batch Cooking and Freezing

1. **Time Efficiency**

- Cooking in large quantities reduces the need for daily meal preparation, freeing up time for other activities and rest.

2. **Consistency**
   - Ensures that nutritious meals are always available, supporting a balanced diet and aiding recovery.
3. **Cost Savings**
   - Buying ingredients in bulk and reducing food waste can lower overall food costs.
4. **Portion Control**
   - Pre-portioning meals helps manage portion sizes and calorie intake, which is important for weight management and overall health.

Planning and Preparation

1. **Create a Meal Plan**
   - Plan meals for a week or more, focusing on dishes that freeze well. Consider breakfast, lunch, dinner, and snacks.

2. **Make a Shopping List**

- List all ingredients needed for the planned meals and shop in bulk to save time and money.

3. **Organize the Kitchen**
   - Ensure you have enough storage containers, freezer bags, and labels. Clear space in the freezer to accommodate the batch-cooked meals.

Best Practices for Batch Cooking

1. **Choose Freezer-Friendly Recipes**
   - Opt for meals that retain their texture and flavor after freezing, such as soups, stews, casseroles, and pasta dishes.
2. **Double or Triple Recipes**
   - Cook larger quantities of recipes, ensuring you have enough to freeze for future use.
3. **Cook in Stages**
   - Prepare different components (e.g., proteins, grains, vegetables) separately and combine them into meals later. This can also allow for more variety.
4. **Cool Before Freezing**
   - Let cooked foods cool to room temperature before freezing to prevent freezer burn and preserve texture.

Tips for Freezing Meals

1. **Use Proper Containers**
   - Select freezer-safe containers or bags. Glass containers with airtight lids, BPA-free plastic containers, and heavy-duty freezer bags work well.
2. **Portion Control**
   - Divide meals into individual or family-sized portions to make reheating easier and to prevent waste.
3. **Label Clearly**
   - Label each container or bag with the meal name and the date it was frozen. Include reheating instructions if needed.
4. **Remove Air**
   - When using freezer bags, remove as much air as possible to prevent freezer burn. Vacuum sealing is an excellent option if available.

Sample Batch Cooking Plan

Week 1:

1. **Breakfast**
   - **Oatmeal Cups**: Prepare baked oatmeal cups with fruits and nuts.

Freeze individually and reheat in the
microwave.

- ○ **Smoothie Packs**: Assemble freezer
  packs with fruits, greens, and seeds.
  Blend with liquid when ready to eat.

2. **Lunch**
   - ○ **Quinoa and Vegetable Bowls**: Cook
     quinoa and roast vegetables. Portion
     into containers with a protein
     (chicken, tofu, beans) and a dressing
     on the side.
   - ○ **Lentil Soup**: Make a large pot of lentil
     soup. Cool, portion into containers,
     and freeze.

3. **Dinner**
   - ○ **Chicken and Vegetable Stir-Fry**:
     Cook a large batch of stir-fry and
     freeze in meal-sized portions.
   - ○ **Baked Ziti**: Prepare a large dish of
     baked ziti. Divide into portions and
     freeze.

4. **Snacks**
   - ○ **Energy Balls**: Make a batch of energy
     balls with oats, nuts, and dried fruit.
     Freeze and take out as needed.
   - ○ **Vegetable Sticks and Hummus**: Pre-
     cut vegetables and portion hummus
     into containers. Freeze hummus in ice
     cube trays for portion control.

Week 2:

1. **Breakfast**
   - **Egg Muffins**: Bake egg muffins with vegetables and cheese. Freeze and reheat in the microwave.
   - **Whole Grain Pancakes**: Make a large batch of pancakes. Cool, separate with parchment paper, and freeze.
2. **Lunch**
   - **Chili**: Cook a large pot of chili. Cool, portion, and freeze.
   - **Chicken Salad Wraps**: Prepare chicken salad, portion into containers, and freeze the filling. Use fresh wraps.
3. **Dinner**
   - **Beef Stew**: Make a large batch of beef stew. Cool, portion, and freeze.
   - **Vegetable Lasagna**: Prepare vegetable lasagna, portion, and freeze.
4. **Snacks**
   - **Fruit and Yogurt Parfaits**: Layer fruit and yogurt in containers. Freeze and thaw in the fridge overnight before eating.
   - **Homemade Granola Bars**: Make granola bars, cut into portions, and freeze.

Reheating and Serving

1. **Thawing**
   - Thaw meals in the refrigerator overnight or use the defrost setting on the microwave.
2. **Reheating**
   - Reheat meals on the stovetop, in the oven, or in the microwave until they reach the desired temperature. Stir occasionally for even heating.
3. **Serving**
   - Pair frozen meals with fresh sides like salads or steamed vegetables to add variety and freshness.

Safety Tips

1. **Proper Cooling**
   - Cool cooked foods quickly to room temperature before freezing to prevent bacterial growth.
2. **Storage Time**
   - Most frozen meals are best consumed within 2-3 months. Label with dates to track storage time.
3. **Avoid Refreezing**
   - Do not refreeze meals that have been thawed to ensure food safety and quality.

Batch cooking and freezing meals can significantly ease the burden of daily meal preparation for stroke patients and their caregivers. By planning ahead and using these tips, nutritious and delicious meals are always within reach, supporting recovery and overall well-being.

Chapter 5

5.1 Breakfast Options

Breakfast is an important meal for stroke recovery, providing essential nutrients and energy to start the day. Here are some nutritious and easy-to-prepare breakfast options:

Quick and Nutritious Breakfast Ideas

1. **Oatmeal with Fresh Fruit and Nuts**
   - **Ingredients**: Rolled oats, milk (or plant-based milk), fresh berries, sliced banana, nuts (such as almonds or walnuts), honey or maple syrup (optional).
   - **Preparation**: Cook oats according to package instructions. Top with fresh fruits, nuts, and a drizzle of honey or maple syrup.
2. **Greek Yogurt Parfait**
   - **Ingredients**: Greek yogurt, granola, mixed berries (such as strawberries, blueberries, raspberries), honey or agave syrup (optional).
   - **Preparation**: Layer Greek yogurt, granola, and berries in a glass or bowl.

Drizzle with honey or agave syrup if desired.

3. **Smoothies**
   - **Ingredients**: Spinach or kale, frozen mixed berries, banana, Greek yogurt or protein powder, almond milk or juice.
   - **Preparation**: Blend all ingredients until smooth. Add more liquid as needed for desired consistency.

4. **Whole Grain Toast with Avocado**
   - **Ingredients**: Whole grain bread, ripe avocado, cherry tomatoes, salt, pepper, olive oil (optional).
   - **Preparation**: Toast whole grain bread. Spread mashed avocado on top. Season with salt and pepper. Serve with sliced cherry tomatoes. Drizzle with olive oil if desired.

5. **Egg and Vegetable Scramble**
   - **Ingredients**: Eggs, bell peppers, spinach, cherry tomatoes, olive oil, salt, pepper, whole grain toast (optional).
   - **Preparation**: Heat olive oil in a pan. Add chopped vegetables and sauté until tender. Whisk eggs and pour over vegetables. Cook until eggs are set. Serve with whole grain toast if desired.

6. **Chia Seed Pudding**
   - **Ingredients**: Chia seeds, milk (or plant-based milk), vanilla extract, honey or maple syrup, fresh fruit (such as berries or mango).
   - **Preparation**: Mix chia seeds, milk, vanilla extract, and sweetener in a bowl or jar. Refrigerate overnight or for at least 2 hours until thickened. Top with fresh fruit before serving.
7. **Whole Grain Pancakes**
   - **Ingredients**: Whole grain pancake mix (or homemade batter), fresh berries, Greek yogurt, honey or maple syrup.
   - **Preparation**: Prepare pancake batter according to package instructions. Cook pancakes on a griddle until golden brown. Serve with fresh berries, Greek yogurt, and a drizzle of honey or maple syrup.
8. **Cottage Cheese with Fruit**
   - **Ingredients**: Cottage cheese, pineapple chunks, mango slices, kiwi slices, honey (optional).
   - **Preparation**: Arrange cottage cheese in a bowl. Top with fresh fruit. Drizzle with honey if desired.

Tips for Breakfast Preparation

- **Prep Ahead**: Prepare ingredients or assemble components (like overnight oats or smoothie packs) the night before to save time in the morning.
- **Balance Nutrients**: Include a combination of carbohydrates (whole grains, fruits), proteins (dairy, eggs, yogurt), and healthy fats (nuts, seeds, avocado) for a balanced meal.
- **Hydrate**: Start the day with a glass of water or herbal tea to stay hydrated.
- **Portion Control**: Measure ingredients to manage calorie intake and ensure balanced nutrition.

These breakfast options provide a variety of flavors and nutrients essential for stroke recovery, supporting overall health and energy levels throughout the day.

5.2 Lunch Ideas

Lunch is an important meal that should be nutritious and satisfying, providing essential nutrients to support recovery and overall health.

Here are some healthy and easy-to-prepare lunch ideas:

Nutritious and Easy Lunch Options

1. **Quinoa Salad with Chickpeas and Vegetables**
   - **Ingredients**: Quinoa, cherry tomatoes, cucumber, red onion, chickpeas, feta cheese (optional), lemon vinaigrette.
   - **Preparation**: Cook quinoa according to package instructions. Toss with chopped vegetables, chickpeas, and feta cheese. Drizzle with lemon vinaigrette.
2. **Chicken and Vegetable Stir-Fry**
   - **Ingredients**: Chicken breast, bell peppers, broccoli, snap peas, soy sauce, garlic, ginger, brown rice.
   - **Preparation**: Stir-fry chicken until cooked through. Add vegetables and sauté until tender-crisp. Season with soy sauce, garlic, and ginger. Serve over brown rice.
3. **Turkey and Avocado Wrap**
   - **Ingredients**: Whole grain tortilla wrap, sliced turkey breast, avocado, lettuce, tomato, mustard or hummus.
   - **Preparation**: Spread mustard or hummus on the tortilla. Layer with

turkey slices, avocado, lettuce, and
tomato. Roll up tightly and slice in
half.

4. **Vegetable and Lentil Soup**
   - **Ingredients**: Lentils, carrots, celery,
     onion, garlic, vegetable broth, diced
     tomatoes, spinach, herbs (such as
     thyme and bay leaves).
   - **Preparation**: Sauté onion, garlic,
     carrots, and celery in a pot until
     softened. Add lentils, diced tomatoes,
     vegetable broth, and herbs. Simmer
     until lentils are tender. Stir in spinach
     before serving.

5. **Salmon and Quinoa Bowl**
   - **Ingredients**: Grilled or baked salmon
     fillet, quinoa, mixed greens, avocado
     slices, cherry tomatoes, lemon-dill
     dressing.
   - **Preparation**: Cook quinoa according
     to package instructions. Arrange
     mixed greens in a bowl. Top with
     quinoa, grilled salmon, avocado slices,
     and cherry tomatoes. Drizzle with
     lemon-dill dressing.

6. **Greek Chickpea Salad**
   - **Ingredients**: Chickpeas, cucumber,
     cherry tomatoes, red onion, Kalamata
     olives, feta cheese, lemon vinaigrette.

- **Preparation**: Combine chickpeas, chopped vegetables, olives, and feta cheese in a bowl. Toss with lemon vinaigrette.

7. **Tuna Salad Stuffed Bell Peppers**
   - **Ingredients**: Bell peppers, canned tuna, celery, red onion, Greek yogurt, lemon juice, Dijon mustard, parsley.
   - **Preparation**: Cut bell peppers in half and remove seeds. Mix tuna with celery, red onion, Greek yogurt, lemon juice, Dijon mustard, and parsley. Stuff mixture into bell pepper halves.

8. **Mediterranean Couscous Salad**
   - **Ingredients**: Whole wheat couscous, cucumber, cherry tomatoes, red bell pepper, olives, feta cheese, lemon-herb dressing.
   - **Preparation**: Cook couscous according to package instructions. Toss with chopped vegetables, olives, and feta cheese. Drizzle with lemon-herb dressing.

Tips for Lunch Preparation

- **Prepare Ahead**: Cook grains, proteins, and dressings in advance to assemble lunches quickly during the week.
- **Balance Nutrients**: Include a combination of lean proteins, whole grains, healthy fats (like avocado or olive oil), and plenty of vegetables for fiber and vitamins.
- **Portion Control**: Use meal prep containers to portion out lunches ahead of time for easy grab-and-go meals.
- **Hydrate**: Enjoy water or herbal tea with lunch to stay hydrated throughout the day.

These lunch ideas are designed to be nutritious, flavorful, and convenient, making them ideal for supporting stroke recovery and maintaining overall health.

5.3 Dinner Recipes

Dinner is an opportunity to enjoy a nutritious and satisfying meal that supports recovery and overall health. Here are some wholesome and easy-to-prepare dinner recipes:

Wholesome Dinner Ideas

1. **Grilled Lemon Herb Chicken with Roasted Vegetables**
   - **Ingredients**: Chicken breasts, lemon zest, garlic, thyme, rosemary, olive oil, bell peppers, zucchini, red onion.
   - **Preparation**: Marinate chicken breasts in lemon zest, garlic, thyme, rosemary, and olive oil. Grill until cooked through. Serve with roasted vegetables.
2. **Baked Salmon with Quinoa and Steamed Broccoli**
   - **Ingredients**: Salmon fillets, lemon juice, dill, olive oil, quinoa, broccoli.
   - **Preparation**: Season salmon with lemon juice, dill, and olive oil. Bake until flaky. Serve with cooked quinoa and steamed broccoli.
3. **Vegetable and Bean Chili**
   - **Ingredients**: Kidney beans, black beans, diced tomatoes, bell peppers, onion, garlic, chili powder, cumin, paprika.
   - **Preparation**: Sauté onion, garlic, and bell peppers until softened. Add beans, diced tomatoes, and spices. Simmer until flavors meld. Serve hot.

4. **Turkey Meatballs with Whole Wheat Pasta**
    - **Ingredients**: Ground turkey, whole wheat breadcrumbs, egg, Parmesan cheese, garlic, marinara sauce, whole wheat pasta.
    - **Preparation**: Mix ground turkey with breadcrumbs, egg, Parmesan cheese, and garlic. Form into meatballs and bake until cooked through. Serve with whole wheat pasta and marinara sauce.
5. **Stir-Fried Tofu with Vegetables**
    - **Ingredients**: Extra-firm tofu, bell peppers, snap peas, carrots, soy sauce, garlic, ginger, sesame oil, brown rice.
    - **Preparation**: Press tofu to remove excess moisture and cut into cubes. Stir-fry with vegetables, garlic, and ginger until tender. Add soy sauce and sesame oil. Serve over brown rice.
6. **Quinoa Stuffed Bell Peppers**
    - **Ingredients**: Bell peppers, quinoa, black beans, corn, cherry tomatoes, cilantro, cumin, chili powder, salsa.
    - **Preparation**: Cook quinoa according to package instructions. Mix with black beans, corn, cherry tomatoes, cilantro, cumin, and chili powder. Stuff mixture into halved bell peppers.

Bake until peppers are tender. Serve with salsa.

7. **Pesto Pasta with Chicken and Roasted Vegetables**
   - **Ingredients**: Whole wheat pasta, chicken breast, pesto sauce, cherry tomatoes, spinach, Parmesan cheese.
   - **Preparation**: Cook pasta according to package instructions. Grill or sauté chicken until cooked through. Toss pasta with pesto sauce, cherry tomatoes, spinach, and grilled chicken. Sprinkle with Parmesan cheese before serving.

8. **Vegetable and Lentil Curry**
   - **Ingredients**: Red lentils, onion, garlic, ginger, curry powder, coconut milk, spinach, cauliflower, peas.
   - **Preparation**: Sauté onion, garlic, and ginger until fragrant. Add curry powder and cook briefly. Stir in red lentils and coconut milk. Simmer until lentils are tender. Add spinach, cauliflower, and peas. Cook until vegetables are tender. Serve hot.

Tips for Dinner Preparation

- **Prep Ahead**: Chop vegetables, marinate proteins, and cook grains ahead of time to streamline dinner preparation.
- **Balance Nutrients**: Include lean proteins, whole grains or legumes, and plenty of colorful vegetables for a balanced meal.
- **Cooking Methods**: Opt for grilling, baking, or stir-frying with minimal oil to keep meals healthy.
- **Portion Control**: Use smaller plates and bowls to manage portion sizes and prevent overeating.

These dinner recipes are designed to be delicious, nutritious, and supportive of stroke recovery. They incorporate a variety of ingredients to ensure a well-rounded meal that meets nutritional needs and promotes overall health.

5.4 Snacks and Desserts

Snacks and desserts can be enjoyable while also providing essential nutrients to support stroke recovery. Here are some wholesome snack ideas and healthier dessert options:

Wholesome Snack Ideas

1. **Fruit and Nut Mix**
   - **Ingredients**: Mixed nuts (such as almonds, walnuts, and cashews), dried fruits (such as apricots, raisins, and cranberries).
   - **Preparation**: Mix nuts and dried fruits in a container for a convenient grab-and-go snack.
2. **Greek Yogurt with Berries**
   - **Ingredients**: Greek yogurt, fresh berries (such as strawberries, blueberries, raspberries).
   - **Preparation**: Serve Greek yogurt topped with fresh berries for a protein-rich snack.
3. **Vegetable Sticks with Hummus**
   - **Ingredients**: Carrot sticks, celery sticks, cucumber slices, bell pepper strips, hummus.
   - **Preparation**: Dip vegetable sticks into hummus for a crunchy and satisfying snack.
4. **Homemade Energy Bars**
   - **Ingredients**: Rolled oats, nuts (such as almonds or peanuts), dried fruits (such as dates or apricots), honey or maple syrup, nut butter.

- Preparation: Blend oats, nuts, and dried fruits in a food processor. Add honey or maple syrup and nut butter to bind. Press into a pan and refrigerate until firm. Cut into bars.

5. **Whole Grain Crackers with Avocado**
   - **Ingredients**: Whole grain crackers, ripe avocado, lemon juice, salt, pepper.
   - **Preparation**: Spread mashed avocado on whole grain crackers. Season with lemon juice, salt, and pepper.

6. **Smoothies**
   - **Ingredients**: Spinach or kale, frozen mixed berries, banana, Greek yogurt or protein powder, almond milk or juice.
   - **Preparation**: Blend all ingredients until smooth. Add more liquid as needed for desired consistency.

7. **Cottage Cheese with Pineapple**
   - **Ingredients**: Cottage cheese, pineapple chunks.
   - **Preparation**: Serve cottage cheese topped with pineapple chunks for a protein-packed snack.

Healthier Dessert Options

1. **Fruit Salad**

- o **Ingredients**: Mixed fruits (such as strawberries, mangoes, kiwi, and grapes), fresh mint leaves, lemon or lime juice.
  - o **Preparation**: Toss mixed fruits with fresh mint leaves and a squeeze of lemon or lime juice.

2. **Dark Chocolate Covered Almonds**
   - o **Ingredients**: Dark chocolate (70% cocoa or higher), almonds.
   - o **Preparation**: Melt dark chocolate in a microwave or double boiler. Dip almonds into melted chocolate. Place on parchment paper and let cool until chocolate hardens.

3. **Baked Apples with Cinnamon**
   - o **Ingredients**: Apples, cinnamon, honey (optional), nuts (such as walnuts or almonds).
   - o **Preparation**: Core apples and sprinkle with cinnamon. Drizzle with honey if desired. Bake until tender. Serve with chopped nuts on top.

4. **Yogurt Parfait**
   - o **Ingredients**: Greek yogurt, granola, mixed berries (such as strawberries, blueberries, raspberries), honey or agave syrup (optional).
   - o **Preparation**: Layer Greek yogurt, granola, and berries in a glass or bowl.

Drizzle with honey or agave syrup if
desired.

5. **Chia Seed Pudding**
   - **Ingredients**: Chia seeds, milk (or
     plant-based milk), vanilla extract,
     honey or maple syrup, fresh fruit (such
     as berries or mango).
   - **Preparation**: Mix chia seeds, milk,
     vanilla extract, and sweetener in a
     bowl or jar. Refrigerate overnight or
     for at least 2 hours until thickened.
     Top with fresh fruit before serving.

6. **Frozen Banana Bites**
   - **Ingredients**: Bananas, dark chocolate,
     nuts (such as almonds or peanuts),
     shredded coconut (optional).
   - **Preparation**: Slice bananas into
     rounds. Melt dark chocolate and dip
     banana slices into chocolate. Place on
     parchment paper and sprinkle with
     nuts or shredded coconut. Freeze until
     chocolate hardens.

Tips for Snacks and Desserts

- **Portion Control**: Use small bowls or plates
  for snacks and desserts to avoid overeating.
- **Balance Nutrients**: Include a mix of
  carbohydrates, proteins, and healthy fats in
  snacks to keep energy levels stable.

- **Hydration**: Drink water or herbal tea with snacks and desserts to stay hydrated.

These snack and dessert options are designed to be delicious and nutrient-dense, supporting stroke recovery and overall health while satisfying cravings for something sweet or savory.

Chapter 6

6.1 Swallowing Difficulties (Dysphagia)

Dysphagia, or difficulty swallowing, is a common issue faced by stroke patients. Proper nutrition is crucial, but the texture and consistency of food and liquids must be carefully managed to ensure safe swallowing and prevent choking or aspiration. Here are some guidelines and meal ideas to accommodate dysphagia.

Understanding Dysphagia

1. **Causes and Symptoms**
   - **Causes**: Stroke can damage the brain areas responsible for coordinating swallowing.
   - **Symptoms**: Coughing or choking when eating or drinking, a feeling of food stuck in the throat, recurrent pneumonia, and weight loss.
2. **Diagnosis and Management**
   - **Diagnosis**: Conducted by healthcare professionals using swallowing assessments and tests like a videofluoroscopic swallow study.

- Management: Involves dietary modifications, swallowing therapy, and sometimes medical interventions.

Food and Liquid Consistency

1. **Food Texture**
   - **Pureed**: Smooth and uniform, similar to pudding or mashed potatoes.
   - **Minced and Moist**: Finely chopped food moistened with sauces or gravies.
   - **Soft and Bite-Sized**: Soft enough to be easily mashed with a fork.
2. **Liquid Consistency**
   - **Thin Liquids**: Regular liquids like water and juice, may need to be thickened.
   - **Nectar-Thick**: Slightly thickened liquids that flow like nectar.
   - **Honey-Thick**: More thickened, similar to the consistency of honey.
   - **Pudding-Thick**: Very thick, similar to the consistency of pudding.

Nutrition Tips for Dysphagia

1. **Consult a Dietitian**
   - Work with a dietitian to create a personalized meal plan that meets

nutritional needs while considering swallowing difficulties.

2. **Use Thickeners**
    - Commercial thickeners can be added to liquids to achieve the desired consistency.
3. **Small, Frequent Meals**
    - Eating smaller, more frequent meals can help prevent fatigue and make swallowing easier.
4. **Focus on Nutrient-Dense Foods**
    - Ensure that every bite counts by including nutrient-dense foods that provide essential vitamins and minerals.

Sample Meal Ideas for Dysphagia

1. **Breakfast**
    - **Pureed Oatmeal with Banana and Honey**
        - **Ingredients**: Cooked oatmeal, banana, honey.
        - **Preparation**: Blend cooked oatmeal with banana and a small amount of milk until smooth. Sweeten with honey if desired.
    - **Smoothie**

- **Ingredients**: Greek yogurt, blended fruits (such as strawberries, blueberries, and mango), protein powder.
        - **Preparation**: Blend Greek yogurt with fruits and protein powder until smooth. Adjust thickness as needed.

2. **Lunch**
   - **Pureed Chicken and Vegetable Soup**
     - **Ingredients**: Cooked chicken breast, carrots, potatoes, low-sodium chicken broth.
     - **Preparation**: Blend cooked chicken and vegetables with broth until smooth. Heat and serve.

   - **Cottage Cheese with Pureed Peaches**
     - **Ingredients**: Cottage cheese, canned peaches (in natural juice).
     - **Preparation**: Puree canned peaches and serve over cottage cheese.

3. **Dinner**

- **Pureed Meatloaf with Mashed Potatoes and Gravy**
    - **Ingredients**: Cooked meatloaf, mashed potatoes, low-sodium gravy.
    - **Preparation**: Puree meatloaf with gravy until smooth. Serve with smooth mashed potatoes.
- **Minced and Moist Fish with Soft Vegetables**
    - **Ingredients**: Cooked fish fillet, steamed carrots and peas, white sauce.
    - **Preparation**: Finely chop fish and mix with a white sauce to moisten. Serve with mashed carrots and peas.

4. **Snacks and Desserts**
- **Applesauce**
    - **Ingredients**: Apples, cinnamon (optional).
    - **Preparation**: Cook apples until soft, then blend until smooth. Add cinnamon for flavor.
- **Yogurt with Honey**
    - **Ingredients**: Greek yogurt, honey.
    - **Preparation**: Mix Greek yogurt with honey. Ensure the

yogurt is smooth and without chunks.

Tips for Safe Eating and Drinking

1. **Sit Upright**
   - Always sit upright during meals and for at least 30 minutes after eating to help prevent aspiration.

2. **Eat Slowly**
   - Take small bites and sips, and eat slowly to allow adequate time for swallowing.
3. **Avoid Distractions**
   - Minimize distractions during meals to focus on safe swallowing.
4. **Consult a Speech-Language Pathologist (SLP)**
   - Work with an SLP to improve swallowing techniques and learn safe eating strategies.

By carefully managing food and liquid consistency and following these tips, individuals with dysphagia can enjoy safe and nutritious meals that support their recovery and overall well-being.

6.2 Modifying Textures for Safety

For individuals with dysphagia, modifying the texture of foods and liquids is crucial to ensure safe swallowing and prevent choking or aspiration. Here are detailed guidelines on how to modify textures and some practical tips for preparation.

Food Texture Modification

1. **Pureed Foods**
   - **Characteristics**: Smooth, cohesive, and free of lumps.
   - **Preparation Tips**:
     - **Blending**: Use a blender or food processor to achieve a smooth consistency. Add liquids like broth, milk, or water to help achieve the desired texture.
     - **Straining**: After blending, strain foods through a fine sieve to remove any remaining lumps.
   - **Examples**:

- **Pureed Vegetables**: Cooked carrots, peas, or squash blended until smooth.
- **Pureed Meats**: Cooked chicken or beef blended with broth until smooth.
- **Pureed Fruits**: Apples, pears, or bananas blended until smooth.

2. **Minced and Moist Foods**
   - **Characteristics**: Finely chopped to 1/8 inch pieces, moist, and easily formed into a ball with a fork.
   - **Preparation Tips**:
     - **Chopping**: Use a sharp knife or food processor to finely chop foods.
     - **Moistening**: Add sauces, gravies, or broths to keep foods moist.
   - **Examples**:
     - **Minced Meats**: Finely chopped chicken, turkey, or fish with added gravy.
     - **Minced Vegetables**: Finely chopped and cooked vegetables like carrots, peas, or potatoes.
     - **Soft Fruits**: Finely chopped ripe fruits like melons or berries.

3. **Soft and Bite-Sized Foods**
    - **Characteristics**: Soft and easily mashed with a fork, cut into bite-sized pieces.
    - **Preparation Tips**:
        - **Cooking**: Cook foods until very tender.
        - **Cutting**: Cut foods into small, manageable pieces.
    - **Examples**:
        - **Soft Meats**: Tender pieces of chicken, fish, or meatloaf.
        - **Soft Vegetables**: Cooked and tender vegetables like squash, zucchini, or sweet potatoes.
        - **Soft Fruits**: Ripe fruits like bananas, peaches, or mangoes.

Liquid Consistency Modification

1. **Thin Liquids**
    - **Characteristics**: Regular consistency liquids like water, juice, and tea.
    - **Risks**: Thin liquids may pose a high risk of aspiration for some individuals.
    - **Modification**: May need to be thickened to a safer consistency.
2. **Nectar-Thick Liquids**

- o **Characteristics**: Slightly thickened, similar to the consistency of nectar or tomato juice.
- o **Preparation Tips**:
  - ■ **Commercial Thickeners**: Use commercial thickening agents as directed to achieve the desired consistency.
  - ■ **Natural Thickeners**: Add pureed fruits or vegetable juices to thicken naturally.
- o **Examples**:
  - ■ **Thickened Juices**: Orange juice thickened with a commercial thickener.
  - ■ **Smoothies**: Blended fruit smoothies with a thicker consistency.

3. **Honey-Thick Liquids**
   - o **Characteristics**: Thicker than nectar, similar to the consistency of honey.

   - o **Preparation Tips**:
     - ■ **Commercial Thickeners**: Use more thickening agent to achieve the honey-thick consistency.

- **Natural Thickeners**: Pureed fruits or yogurt can be used to thicken drinks.
  - **Examples**:
    - **Thickened Milk**: Milk thickened to honey consistency.
    - **Thickened Soups**: Creamy soups thickened with pureed vegetables or commercial thickeners.

4. **Pudding-Thick Liquids**
   - **Characteristics**: Very thick, similar to the consistency of pudding.
   - **Preparation Tips**:
     - **Commercial Thickeners**: Use a higher concentration of thickening agents.
     - **Natural Thickeners**: Blended puddings or custards can be used.

   - **Examples**:
     - **Pudding**: Prepared pudding cups.
     - **Thickened Desserts**: Yogurt thickened to pudding consistency.

Practical Tips for Safe Texture Modification

1. **Equipment**:
   - **Blenders and Food Processors**: Essential for pureeing foods to the desired consistency.
   - **Sifters and Sieves**: Useful for removing lumps from pureed foods.
   - **Sharp Knives**: Important for finely chopping foods.
2. **Moisture**:
   - **Adding Liquids**: Use broths, gravies, sauces, or water to help achieve the right consistency and keep foods moist.
   - **Prevent Dryness**: Avoid dry foods that can be difficult to swallow.

3. **Flavor and Variety**:
   - **Seasoning**: Use herbs and spices to enhance the flavor of modified foods without adding salt.
   - **Variety**: Offer a variety of foods to ensure a balanced diet and prevent meal fatigue.
4. **Safety First**:

- o **Supervision**: Monitor the individual while eating to ensure safe swallowing.
- o **Consult Professionals**: Regularly consult with speech-language pathologists and dietitians to adjust textures as needed.

By carefully modifying the textures of foods and liquids and following these guidelines, individuals with dysphagia can enjoy safe, nutritious, and enjoyable meals that support their recovery and overall well-being.

6.3 Allergies and Food Intolerances

Managing allergies and food intolerances is crucial for stroke patients to ensure safe and healthy nutrition. Here are some strategies and meal ideas to accommodate common allergies and food intolerances.

Understanding Allergies and Food Intolerances

1. **Food Allergies**

- **Definition**: An immune system reaction that occurs soon after eating a certain food.
    - **Common Allergens**: Peanuts, tree nuts, shellfish, fish, milk, eggs, soy, wheat.
    - **Symptoms**: Hives, swelling, difficulty breathing, anaphylaxis.
2. **Food Intolerances**
    - **Definition**: A digestive system response rather than an immune response.
    - **Common Intolerances**: Lactose, gluten, fructose, sulfites.
    - **Symptoms**: Bloating, gas, diarrhea, stomach pain.

Strategies for Managing Allergies and Intolerances

1. **Label Reading**
    - Carefully read food labels to identify potential allergens or intolerant ingredients.
2. **Avoid Cross-Contamination**
    - Use separate utensils, cookware, and preparation areas for allergen-free foods.
3. **Substitute Ingredients**

- Replace allergenic ingredients with safe alternatives. For example, use almond milk instead of cow's milk.

4. **Consult Healthcare Providers**
   - Work with dietitians and healthcare providers to create a personalized meal plan that avoids allergens and intolerant foods.

5. **Food Allergy Action Plan**
   - Have a plan in place for managing accidental exposure, including emergency medication like epinephrine.

Allergy-Friendly Meal Ideas

1. **Breakfast**
   - **Dairy-Free Smoothie**
     - **Ingredients**: Almond milk, frozen berries, banana, spinach.
     - **Preparation**: Blend all ingredients until smooth.
   - **Gluten-Free Oatmeal**
     - **Ingredients**: Gluten-free oats, almond milk, fresh fruit, honey.
     - **Preparation**: Cook oats in almond milk. Top with fresh fruit and honey.

2. **Lunch**
   - **Nut-Free Quinoa Salad**

- **Ingredients**: Quinoa, cherry tomatoes, cucumber, bell peppers, olive oil, lemon juice.
- **Preparation**: Cook quinoa according to package instructions. Toss with chopped vegetables, olive oil, and lemon juice.

- **Egg-Free Chickpea Salad Sandwich**
  - **Ingredients**: Canned chickpeas, avocado, lemon juice, whole grain bread.
  - **Preparation**: Mash chickpeas and avocado together. Season with lemon juice and spread on bread.

3. **Dinner**
   - **Gluten-Free Pasta with Tomato and Basil**
     - **Ingredients**: Gluten-free pasta, cherry tomatoes, fresh basil, olive oil, garlic.
     - **Preparation**: Cook pasta according to package instructions. Sauté garlic in olive oil, add tomatoes and basil. Toss with pasta.

- ○ **Soy-Free Chicken Stir-Fry**
    - ■ **Ingredients**: Chicken breast, bell peppers, broccoli, carrots, coconut aminos (soy sauce alternative).
    - ■ **Preparation**: Stir-fry chicken and vegetables. Season with coconut aminos.

4. **Snacks**
   - ○ **Fruit and Seed Mix**
     - ■ **Ingredients**: Pumpkin seeds, sunflower seeds, dried cranberries.
     - ■ **Preparation**: Mix all ingredients in a container.
   - ○ **Dairy-Free Yogurt with Berries**
     - ■ **Ingredients**: Coconut yogurt, mixed berries.
     - ■ **Preparation**: Top coconut yogurt with mixed berries.

5. **Desserts**
   - ○ **Lactose-Free Banana Ice Cream**
     - ■ **Ingredients**: Frozen bananas, almond milk.
     - ■ **Preparation**: Blend frozen bananas with almond milk until smooth.
   - ○ **Nut-Free Energy Balls**

- ■ **Ingredients**: Rolled oats, sunflower seed butter, honey, dried fruit.
- ■ **Preparation**: Mix all ingredients and form into balls. Refrigerate until firm.

Tips for Safe Meal Preparation

1. **Dedicated Preparation Area**
   - Designate a separate area for preparing allergen-free meals to prevent cross-contamination.
2. **Clean Utensils and Surfaces**
   - Thoroughly clean all utensils, cutting boards, and surfaces before preparing allergen-free meals.
3. **Education and Awareness**
   - Educate family members and caregivers about the importance of avoiding allergens and recognizing symptoms of an allergic reaction.
4. **Variety and Balance**
   - Ensure meals are balanced and varied to provide all essential nutrients while avoiding allergens or intolerant foods.

By following these guidelines and meal ideas, stroke patients with allergies or food intolerances can enjoy

safe, nutritious, and delicious meals that support
their recovery and overall health.

Chapter 7

7.1 Reading Nutrition Labels

Reading nutrition labels is an essential skill for stroke patients, particularly those managing specific dietary needs such as low sodium, low fat, or allergen-free diets. Understanding how to interpret the information on food labels can help make healthier and safer food choices.

Key Components of a Nutrition Label

1. **Serving Size**
   - **Definition**: Indicates the amount of food that is considered one serving.
   - **Importance**: All the nutritional information on the label is based on this serving size, so it's crucial to compare it to the amount you actually eat.
2. **Calories**
   - **Definition**: The amount of energy provided by one serving of the food.
   - **Importance**: Helps manage daily caloric intake for weight management and overall health.
3. **Nutrients to Limit**

- **Total Fat**: Includes saturated fat and trans fat. Look for low amounts to support heart health.
- **Cholesterol**: Aim for low cholesterol to help manage cardiovascular risk.
- **Sodium**: Essential to monitor for stroke patients, as high sodium can increase blood pressure.
- **Added Sugars**: Limit to reduce the risk of weight gain and other health issues.

4. **Nutrients to Get Enough Of**
   - **Dietary Fiber**: Supports digestive health and can help manage cholesterol levels.
   - **Vitamin D, Calcium, Iron, and Potassium**: Important for bone health, oxygen transport, and overall health.

5. **% Daily Value (%DV)**
   - **Definition**: Shows how much a nutrient in a serving of the food contributes to a daily diet, based on a 2,000-calorie diet.
   - **Importance**: Helps assess whether a serving of food is high or low in a nutrient.
     - **5% DV or less**: Low
     - **20% DV or more**: High

Steps for Reading a Nutrition Label

1. **Check the Serving Size**
   - Compare the serving size to the portion you plan to eat. If you eat double the serving size, you'll need to double the nutrient amounts.
2. **Look at the Calories**
   - Consider how the calories per serving fit into your total daily calorie needs.
3. **Limit Nutrients**
   - Aim for lower %DVs of total fat, saturated fat, trans fat, cholesterol, and sodium.
4. **Get Enough Nutrients**
   - Aim for higher %DVs of dietary fiber, vitamins, and minerals.
5. **Read the Ingredient List**
   - Ingredients are listed in descending order by weight. This can help identify hidden sources of allergens, added sugars, and other ingredients you may want to limit.

Special Considerations for Stroke Patients

1. **Low Sodium**
   - Look for foods labeled as "low sodium" (140 mg or less per serving),

"very low sodium" (35 mg or less per serving), or "salt-free" (less than 5 mg per serving).
  - Avoid foods with high sodium content, such as processed meats, canned soups, and salty snacks.

2. **Low Saturated Fat and Cholesterol**
   - Choose foods with lower amounts of saturated fat and cholesterol. Look for "low-fat" (3 grams or less per serving) and "cholesterol-free" (less than 2 mg per serving) options.

3. **High Fiber**
   - Aim for foods high in dietary fiber to support heart health and digestion. Look for products labeled "high fiber" (5 grams or more per serving).

4. **Allergens**
   - Carefully check the ingredient list for any allergens. Common allergens include milk, eggs, fish, shellfish, tree nuts, peanuts, wheat, and soybeans.

Practical Examples

1. **Canned Soup Label Analysis**
   - **Serving Size**: 1 cup (245 grams)

- o **Calories**: 100 per serving
- o **Total Fat**: 2 grams (3% DV)
- o **Sodium**: 800 mg (35% DV) – High; choose lower-sodium options or make homemade soup.
- o **Dietary Fiber**: 2 grams (8% DV)
- o **Protein**: 3 grams
- o **Vitamins and Minerals**: Check for calcium, iron, and other nutrients.

2. **Breakfast Cereal Label Analysis**
   - o **Serving Size**: 1 cup (30 grams)
   - o **Calories**: 120 per serving
   - o **Total Fat**: 1 gram (1% DV)
   - o **Sodium**: 200 mg (9% DV)
   - o **Dietary Fiber**: 4 grams (16% DV) – High; good choice.
   - o **Sugars**: 10 grams – Consider a lower-sugar option.
   - o **Vitamins and Minerals**: Check for fortification with vitamins and minerals like iron and calcium.

By following these steps and understanding the key components of nutrition labels, stroke patients can make informed choices that align with their dietary needs and health goals.

7.2 Choosing Fresh and Whole Foods

Incorporating fresh and whole foods into the diet is crucial for stroke recovery. These foods are rich in essential nutrients, free from harmful additives, and contribute to overall health and well-being. Here are some tips and guidelines for choosing the best fresh and whole foods.

Benefits of Fresh and Whole Foods

1. **Nutrient Density**
   - Fresh and whole foods are typically more nutrient-dense than processed foods, providing essential vitamins, minerals, and antioxidants.
2. **Fewer Additives**
   - These foods contain fewer additives, preservatives, and artificial ingredients, reducing exposure to potentially harmful substances.
3. **Better Digestion**
   - Whole foods often contain more fiber, which aids in digestion and helps regulate blood sugar levels.
4. **Improved Heart Health**
   - Fresh fruits, vegetables, and whole grains support cardiovascular health by reducing cholesterol levels and blood pressure.

Tips for Choosing Fresh and Whole Foods

1. **Shop the Perimeter of the Grocery Store**
    - The outer edges of the store typically contain fresh produce, meats, dairy, and other whole foods. Avoid the inner aisles where processed foods are usually found.
2. **Select Seasonal Produce**
    - Seasonal fruits and vegetables are often fresher, more flavorful, and more nutritious. They are also generally more affordable.
3. **Read Labels Carefully**
    - For packaged whole foods, such as frozen vegetables or whole grain products, check the ingredient list to ensure no added sugars, sodium, or preservatives.
4. **Buy Organic When Possible**
    - Organic foods are grown without synthetic pesticides and fertilizers, reducing exposure to harmful chemicals. Prioritize organic options for the "Dirty Dozen" - a list of produce with the highest pesticide residues.
5. **Prioritize Variety**

- Include a variety of colors and types of fruits, vegetables, and whole grains to ensure a wide range of nutrients.

Choosing Specific Fresh and Whole Foods

1. **Fruits and Vegetables**
    - **Color and Firmness**: Choose vibrant, firm produce without bruises or blemishes.
    - **Seasonal Selections**: Prioritize seasonal fruits and vegetables for peak freshness and nutrition.
    - **Storage**: Store properly to maintain freshness; for example, refrigerate berries and leafy greens, and keep root vegetables in a cool, dark place.
2. **Whole Grains**
    - **Types**: Brown rice, quinoa, oats, barley, and whole wheat products.
    - **Label Check**: Ensure "whole grain" is listed as the first ingredient and avoid products with added sugars or refined grains.
3. **Lean Proteins**
    - **Sources**: Skinless poultry, fish, lean cuts of beef and pork, eggs, legumes, and tofu.

o **Quality**: Choose fresh, unprocessed meats and opt for wild-caught fish when possible.
o **Preparation**: Prepare using healthy methods like grilling, baking, or steaming.

4. **Dairy and Dairy Alternatives**
   o **Options**: Low-fat or fat-free milk, yogurt, and cheese; plant-based milks like almond, soy, or oat milk.
   o **Label Check**: Look for products with minimal added sugars and artificial ingredients.

5. **Nuts and Seeds**
   o **Types**: Almonds, walnuts, chia seeds, flaxseeds, pumpkin seeds.
   o **Quality**: Choose raw or dry-roasted options without added salt or sugar.

Practical Tips for Incorporating Fresh and Whole Foods

1. **Meal Planning**
   o Plan meals around whole foods to ensure a balanced diet and avoid the temptation of processed foods.
   o **Example**: Plan a week of dinners using seasonal vegetables, lean proteins, and whole grains.

2. **Batch Cooking**

o   Prepare large quantities of whole foods like grains, beans, and roasted vegetables to have on hand for quick meals.

3. **Healthy Snacks**
    o   Keep fresh fruit, cut vegetables, nuts, and yogurt available for easy and nutritious snacks.

4. **Cooking Methods**
    o   Use healthy cooking methods such as steaming, grilling, baking, and roasting to preserve nutrients and enhance flavors without added fats or sodium.

5. **Mindful Eating**
    o   Focus on the quality and enjoyment of whole foods, paying attention to hunger and fullness cues.

Example Meal Ideas

1. **Breakfast**
    o   **Oatmeal with Fresh Berries and Nuts**
        ▪   **Ingredients**: Rolled oats, almond milk, fresh berries, chopped nuts.

- **Preparation**: Cook oats in almond milk, top with berries and nuts.
- **Green Smoothie**
    - **Ingredients**: Spinach, banana, frozen mango, Greek yogurt, water.
    - **Preparation**: Blend all ingredients until smooth.

2. **Lunch**
    - **Quinoa and Black Bean Salad**
        - **Ingredients**: Cooked quinoa, black beans, cherry tomatoes, corn, avocado, lime juice.
        - **Preparation**: Mix all ingredients together and dress with lime juice.
    - **Grilled Chicken and Vegetable Wrap**
        - **Ingredients**: Whole wheat tortilla, grilled chicken breast, mixed greens, sliced bell peppers, hummus.
        - **Preparation**: Spread hummus on the tortilla, add chicken and vegetables, and wrap.

3. **Dinner**
    - **Baked Salmon with Roasted Vegetables**

- **Ingredients**: Salmon fillet, olive oil, lemon, assorted vegetables (such as carrots, broccoli, and bell peppers).
- **Preparation**: Bake salmon with a drizzle of olive oil and lemon. Roast vegetables with olive oil and seasonings.
  - **Stir-Fry with Tofu and Brown Rice**
    - **Ingredients**: Firm tofu, mixed vegetables (such as broccoli, snap peas, carrots), brown rice, low-sodium soy sauce.
    - **Preparation**: Stir-fry tofu and vegetables, serve over brown rice, and season with soy sauce.

4. **Snacks**
   - **Apple Slices with Almond Butter**
     - **Ingredients**: Fresh apple, almond butter.
     - **Preparation**: Slice apple and serve with almond butter for dipping.
   - **Greek Yogurt with Honey and Chia Seeds**
     - **Ingredients**: Plain Greek yogurt, honey, chia seeds.
     - **Preparation**: Mix honey and chia seeds into yogurt.

By prioritizing fresh and whole foods, stroke patients can support their recovery and overall health with nutrient-rich, delicious meals.

7.3 Budget-Friendly Shopping Tips

Maintaining a healthy diet on a budget is entirely possible with some strategic planning and smart shopping habits. Here are some tips for stroke patients and caregivers to buy nutritious foods without breaking the bank.

Plan Ahead

1. **Meal Planning**
   - **Weekly Menus**: Plan your meals for the week based on what's on sale and what you already have in your pantry.
   - **Ingredient List**: Make a shopping list of ingredients needed for your planned meals to avoid impulse buys.

2. **Use Circulars and Coupons**
   - **Sales Flyers**: Check grocery store circulars for weekly sales and discounts.
   - **Coupons**: Use coupons from newspapers, online, or store apps to save on groceries.
3. **Budget-Friendly Recipes**
   - **Choose Inexpensive Ingredients**: Incorporate more budget-friendly staples like beans, lentils, eggs, and in-season vegetables.
   - **One-Pot Meals**: Simplify cooking and save money by preparing one-pot dishes that use fewer ingredients.

Shop Smart

1. **Buy in Bulk**
   - **Dry Goods**: Purchase items like rice, oats, pasta, beans, and lentils in bulk.
   - **Freezing**: Buy larger quantities of meat and fish when on sale and freeze in portions.

2. **Generic Brands**
   - **Store Brands**: Opt for store brands or generic products, which are often

cheaper but similar in quality to name brands.

3. **Choose Whole Foods**
   - **Less Processed**: Whole foods like fresh produce, bulk grains, and lean meats are often cheaper and healthier than processed foods.

4. **Seasonal Produce**
   - **In-Season**: Buy fruits and vegetables that are in season as they are often less expensive and more nutritious.
   - **Farmers' Markets**: Visit local farmers' markets for fresh, affordable produce.

5. **Frozen and Canned Options**
   - **Frozen Vegetables and Fruits**: These can be less expensive and just as nutritious as fresh, with a longer shelf life.
   - **Canned Goods**: Opt for low-sodium canned vegetables and fruits packed in water or their own juice.

Cook Efficiently

1. **Batch Cooking**
   - **Cook in Bulk**: Prepare large batches of meals and freeze portions for future use.

- **Soups and Stews**: Make big pots of soups, stews, and casseroles that can be stretched over multiple meals.

2. **Use Leftovers**
   - **Repurpose Meals**: Get creative with leftovers by turning them into new dishes (e.g., roasted vegetables in salads or frittatas).

3. **Simple Recipes**
   - **Easy Meals**: Stick to recipes with few ingredients and minimal preparation time to save money and effort.

Healthy and Affordable Food Choices

1. **Proteins**
   - **Eggs**: Inexpensive and versatile, great for breakfast, lunch, or dinner.
   - **Chicken Thighs and Drumsticks**: Cheaper than chicken breasts and just as nutritious.
   - **Beans and Lentils**: Cost-effective sources of protein and fiber.
   - **Canned Tuna and Salmon**: Affordable alternatives to fresh fish, rich in omega-3 fatty acids.

2. **Grains**
   - **Brown Rice**: Nutritious and filling, often cheaper when bought in bulk.

o **Whole Grain Pasta**: Affordable and healthier than refined pasta.
   o **Oats**: A versatile and inexpensive option for breakfast and baking.
3. **Vegetables**
   o **Carrots, Potatoes, and Onions**: Cheap, long-lasting, and versatile.
   o **Cabbage and Spinach**: Affordable leafy greens that can be used in various dishes.
   o **Frozen Vegetables**: Budget-friendly and convenient.
4. **Fruits**
   o **Bananas**: Inexpensive and rich in potassium.
   o **Apples**: Long-lasting and versatile.
   o **Frozen Berries**: Cost-effective alternative to fresh berries, great for smoothies and baking.

Example Budget-Friendly Meal Plan

1. **Breakfast**
   o **Overnight Oats**
      ▪ **Ingredients**: Rolled oats, milk or milk alternative, honey, banana.
      ▪ **Preparation**: Mix oats with milk and honey, top with sliced

banana, and refrigerate overnight.

- **Vegetable Omelet**
  - **Ingredients**: Eggs, mixed vegetables (like spinach, onions, and bell peppers).
  - **Preparation**: Sauté vegetables, add beaten eggs, and cook until set.

2. **Lunch**
   - **Lentil Soup**
     - **Ingredients**: Lentils, carrots, onions, celery, canned tomatoes, broth.
     - **Preparation**: Sauté vegetables, add lentils and broth, simmer until lentils are tender.
   - **Quinoa Salad**
     - **Ingredients**: Cooked quinoa, canned chickpeas, cucumber, tomato, olive oil, lemon juice.
     - **Preparation**: Mix cooked quinoa with chickpeas and chopped vegetables, dress with olive oil and lemon juice.

3. **Dinner**
   - **Chicken and Vegetable Stir-Fry**
     - **Ingredients**: Chicken thighs, mixed vegetables (like broccoli,

carrots, bell peppers), soy
sauce, rice.
- **Preparation**: Stir-fry chicken
  and vegetables, serve over
  cooked rice.
- **Bean and Rice Burritos**
  - **Ingredients**: Brown rice, black
    beans, canned corn, salsa,
    whole wheat tortillas.
  - **Preparation**: Cook rice, mix
    with beans and corn, wrap in
    tortillas with salsa.

4. **Snacks**
   - **Fruit and Nut Mix**
     - **Ingredients**: Mixed nuts, dried
       fruit (like raisins or
       cranberries).
     - **Preparation**: Mix and portion
       into snack bags.
   - **Veggie Sticks with Hummus**
     - **Ingredients**: Carrot sticks,
       cucumber slices, store-bought
       or homemade hummus.
     - **Preparation**: Cut vegetables
       and serve with hummus.

By implementing these budget-friendly shopping
and meal preparation tips, stroke patients and their

caregivers can ensure they are eating healthily without overspending.

Chapter 8

8.1 Low-Fat Cooking Methods

Adopting low-fat cooking methods can significantly contribute to a healthier diet, particularly for stroke patients who need to manage their cardiovascular health. Here are some effective and practical low-fat cooking techniques to help reduce fat intake while still enjoying delicious and nutritious meals.

Steaming

1. **Description**: Cooking food using steam from boiling water.
2. **Benefits**: Preserves nutrients, adds no fat, and keeps food moist.
3. **Suitable Foods**: Vegetables, fish, poultry, and dumplings.
4. **Tips**:
    - Use a steamer basket or a steam oven.
    - Season with herbs, spices, or a splash of lemon juice before steaming.

Grilling

1. **Description**: Cooking food on a grill over direct heat.
2. **Benefits**: Allows fat to drip away from the food, resulting in lower fat content.
3. **Suitable Foods**: Lean meats, fish, vegetables, and fruits.
4. **Tips**:
   - Use a grill pan or outdoor grill.
   - Marinate meats to enhance flavor and prevent drying out.
   - Use lean cuts and trim visible fat.

Broiling

1. **Description**: Cooking food under direct heat.
2. **Benefits**: Similar to grilling, allows fat to drip away and cooks quickly.
3. **Suitable Foods**: Fish, lean meats, and vegetables.
4. **Tips**:
   - Place food on a broiler pan to catch drippings.
   - Keep an eye on the food to prevent burning.

Baking

1. **Description**: Cooking food using dry heat in an oven.

2. **Benefits**: Requires minimal added fat.
3. **Suitable Foods**: Meats, fish, vegetables, and casseroles.
4. **Tips**:
   - Use non-stick bakeware or line with parchment paper to reduce the need for oil.
   - Experiment with low-fat marinades and rubs for added flavor.

Roasting

1. **Description**: Cooking food using dry heat in an oven, often at high temperatures.
2. **Benefits**: Enhances the natural flavors of food with minimal added fat.
3. **Suitable Foods**: Vegetables, poultry, and lean meats.
4. **Tips**:
   - Use a rack to allow fat to drip away.
   - Toss vegetables with a small amount of olive oil and seasonings.

Poaching

1. **Description**: Cooking food gently in simmering liquid.
2. **Benefits**: Adds no fat and keeps food tender.
3. **Suitable Foods**: Eggs, fish, chicken, and fruits.

4. **Tips**:
    - Use broth, water, or a mix of water and wine.
    - Add aromatics like herbs, spices, and citrus to the poaching liquid for flavor.

Sautéing

1. **Description**: Cooking food quickly in a small amount of oil over medium-high heat.
2. **Benefits**: Uses less fat compared to frying and retains flavor and nutrients.
3. **Suitable Foods**: Vegetables, lean meats, and seafood.
4. **Tips**:
    - Use a non-stick skillet to reduce the amount of oil needed.
    - Opt for heart-healthy oils like olive or canola oil and use sparingly.

Stir-Frying

1. **Description**: Cooking food quickly in a small amount of oil at high heat, typically in a wok.
2. **Benefits**: Uses minimal oil and preserves the texture and nutrients of the food.
3. **Suitable Foods**: Vegetables, lean meats, tofu, and shrimp.
4. **Tips**:
    - Use a non-stick wok or skillet.

- o Prepare all ingredients before starting as the cooking process is fast.
  - o Use a small amount of oil and avoid heavy sauces.

Microwaving

1. **Description**: Cooking food using microwave radiation.
2. **Benefits**: Quick, convenient, and requires no added fat.
3. **Suitable Foods**: Vegetables, fish, and reheating leftovers.
4. **Tips**:
   - o Use microwave-safe containers.
   - o Add a splash of water or broth to vegetables to steam them.
   - o Cover food to retain moisture.

Using Healthy Substitutes

1. **Dairy Substitutes**
   - o Use low-fat or non-fat versions of milk, yogurt, and cheese.
   - o Replace cream with evaporated skim milk or Greek yogurt.
2. **Oil Substitutes**
   - o Use applesauce or mashed bananas in baking recipes to replace oil or butter.

- o Choose cooking sprays or brush oil lightly on cookware.

3. **Flavor Enhancers**
   - o Use herbs, spices, citrus juices, vinegar, and garlic to add flavor without adding fat.
   - o Experiment with homemade marinades and spice blends.

Example Low-Fat Recipes

1. **Steamed Vegetables**
   - o **Ingredients**: Assorted fresh vegetables (broccoli, carrots, bell peppers), lemon juice, herbs.
   - o **Preparation**: Steam vegetables until tender. Drizzle with lemon juice and sprinkle with herbs before serving.
2. **Grilled Chicken with Vegetables**
   - o **Ingredients**: Skinless chicken breasts, mixed vegetables (zucchini, bell peppers, onions), olive oil, salt, pepper, herbs.
   - o **Preparation**: Marinate chicken with olive oil, salt, pepper, and herbs. Grill chicken and vegetables until cooked through.
3. **Poached Salmon**
   - o **Ingredients**: Salmon fillets, water, lemon slices, dill, peppercorns.

- o **Preparation**: Poach salmon in water with lemon slices, dill, and peppercorns until opaque and flaky.
4. **Stir-Fried Tofu and Vegetables**
   - o **Ingredients**: Firm tofu, mixed vegetables (broccoli, bell peppers, snap peas), low-sodium soy sauce, garlic, ginger.
   - o **Preparation**: Stir-fry tofu and vegetables in a small amount of oil. Add soy sauce, garlic, and ginger for flavor.

By incorporating these low-fat cooking methods, stroke patients can enjoy flavorful, nutritious meals that support their recovery and overall health.

8.2 Reducing Salt without Losing Flavor

Reducing salt intake is essential for stroke patients to manage blood pressure and promote heart health. Fortunately, there are numerous ways to enhance the flavor of food without relying on salt. Here are some strategies and alternatives to help reduce salt while maintaining delicious meals.

Use Herbs and Spices

1. **Herbs**
   - **Fresh and Dried**: Basil, cilantro, parsley, rosemary, thyme, dill, mint, and oregano.
   - **Tips**: Add fresh herbs at the end of cooking to preserve their flavor; dried herbs can be added earlier.
2. **Spices**
   - **Variety**: Cumin, paprika, turmeric, coriander, cinnamon, nutmeg, and cloves.
   - **Tips**: Toast whole spices before grinding them to release their flavors; use a combination of spices for depth.
3. **Blends**
   - **Homemade Mixes**: Create your own salt-free seasoning blends, such as Italian seasoning, curry powder, or chili powder.

Citrus and Vinegars

1. **Citrus**
   - **Options**: Lemon, lime, orange, and grapefruit.

- ○ **Tips**: Use the juice and zest to add brightness and acidity; add citrus just before serving to maintain freshness.

2. **Vinegars**
   - ○ **Varieties**: Balsamic, apple cider, red wine, white wine, and rice vinegar.
   - ○ **Tips**: Use vinegar in marinades, dressings, and as a finishing touch to dishes.

Aromatics and Vegetables

1. **Garlic and Onions**
   - ○ **Forms**: Fresh, roasted, or sautéed.
   - ○ **Tips**: Use garlic and onions to build a flavor base for soups, stews, and sauces.
2. **Ginger and Turmeric**
   - ○ **Forms**: Fresh or ground.
   - ○ **Tips**: Grate fresh ginger or turmeric into stir-fries, soups, and marinades.
3. **Vegetables**
   - ○ **Options**: Mushrooms, bell peppers, tomatoes, and celery.
   - ○ **Tips**: Sauté or roast vegetables to bring out their natural sweetness and depth of flavor.

Umami-Rich Ingredients

1. **Mushrooms**
   - **Types**: Shiitake, portobello, cremini, and button.
   - **Tips**: Use mushrooms to add a savory depth to dishes; consider dried mushrooms for an even stronger flavor.
2. **Tomatoes**
   - **Forms**: Fresh, sun-dried, or tomato paste.
   - **Tips**: Add tomatoes to sauces, soups, and stews for natural umami.
3. **Soy Sauce Alternatives**
   - **Options**: Low-sodium soy sauce, tamari, or coconut aminos.
   - **Tips**: Use sparingly to keep sodium low while adding umami flavor.

Flavorful Liquids

1. **Broths and Stocks**
   - **Types**: Homemade or low-sodium store-bought.
   - **Tips**: Use vegetable, chicken, or beef broth to add depth to soups, stews, and sauces.

2. **Wine and Beer**
    - **Types**: Red and white wine, light beer.
    - **Tips**: Use in cooking to add complexity and richness; alcohol cooks off, leaving the flavor behind.

Fermented Foods

1. **Options**: Kimchi, sauerkraut, miso, and fermented soy products.
2. **Tips**: Use these foods in small amounts to add tangy, savory notes to dishes.

Cooking Techniques

1. **Roasting and Grilling**
    - **Benefits**: Enhances natural flavors through caramelization and browning.
    - **Tips**: Roast or grill vegetables and meats with a light coating of oil and your choice of herbs and spices.
2. **Slow Cooking and Braising**
    - **Benefits**: Develops deep flavors by cooking slowly at low temperatures.
    - **Tips**: Use aromatic vegetables, herbs, and spices to create rich, flavorful dishes without added salt.
3. **Marinating**
    - **Benefits**: Infuses flavors into meats, fish, and vegetables.

- o **Tips**: Use citrus juice, vinegar, herbs, spices, and a small amount of oil for flavorful marinades.

Example Recipes

1. **Herb-Roasted Chicken**
   - o **Ingredients**: Chicken breasts, olive oil, garlic, rosemary, thyme, lemon zest, black pepper.
   - o **Preparation**: Rub chicken with olive oil, garlic, rosemary, thyme, lemon zest, and black pepper. Roast until cooked through.
2. **Citrus-Ginger Stir-Fry**
   - o **Ingredients**: Mixed vegetables (bell peppers, broccoli, snap peas), fresh ginger, garlic, lime juice, low-sodium soy sauce, sesame oil.
   - o **Preparation**: Stir-fry vegetables with ginger and garlic. Add lime juice, soy sauce, and a small amount of sesame oil just before serving.
3. **Mushroom and Tomato Pasta**
   - o **Ingredients**: Whole grain pasta, mixed mushrooms, cherry tomatoes, garlic, balsamic vinegar, basil.
   - o **Preparation**: Sauté mushrooms and garlic, add cherry tomatoes and

balsamic vinegar. Toss with cooked
pasta and fresh basil.
4. **Lemon-Dill Salmon**
   - **Ingredients**: Salmon fillets, lemon
     juice, lemon zest, fresh dill, black
     pepper.
   - **Preparation**: Marinate salmon in
     lemon juice, zest, dill, and pepper.
     Bake or grill until cooked through.

By incorporating these strategies and ingredients,
you can reduce salt without sacrificing flavor,
helping stroke patients maintain a healthy diet and
support their recovery.

8.3 Enhancing Flavor with Herbs and Spices

Herbs and spices are excellent alternatives to salt for
enhancing the flavor of meals, especially beneficial
for stroke patients aiming to reduce sodium intake.
Here's a guide on how to use various herbs and
spices to elevate the taste of dishes while promoting
heart-healthy eating.

Herbs

1. **Basil**
   - **Flavor**: Sweet and slightly peppery.
   - **Uses**: Ideal for pasta dishes, salads, and tomato-based sauces.
2. **Cilantro (Coriander)**
   - **Flavor**: Fresh and citrusy.
   - **Uses**: Common in Mexican, Indian, and Southeast Asian cuisines; adds brightness to salsas and curries.
3. **Parsley**
   - **Flavor**: Clean, slightly peppery.
   - **Uses**: Garnish for soups, salads, and pasta; also used in sauces like chimichurri.
4. **Rosemary**
   - **Flavor**: Pine-like and aromatic.
   - **Uses**: Perfect for roasted meats (especially lamb and chicken), potatoes, and bread.
5. **Thyme**
   - **Flavor**: Earthy and slightly minty.
   - **Uses**: Enhances stews, roasted vegetables, and poultry dishes.
6. **Dill**
   - **Flavor**: Fresh, grassy, and slightly anise-like.

- Uses: Excellent for seafood (like salmon), salads, and yogurt-based sauces.

7. **Mint**
    - **Flavor**: Cool and refreshing.
    - **Uses**: Common in Middle Eastern and Mediterranean dishes, adds flavor to salads, drinks, and desserts.

8. **Oregano**
    - **Flavor**: Robust and slightly bitter.
    - **Uses**: Essential in Italian and Greek cuisines, perfect for pizza, pasta sauces, and grilled meats.

Spices

1. **Cumin**
    - **Flavor**: Warm, earthy, and slightly nutty.
    - **Uses**: Key in Mexican, Indian, and Middle Eastern cuisines; adds depth to chili, curries, and roasted vegetables.

2. **Paprika**
    - **Flavor**: Mildly sweet and smoky.
    - **Uses**: Enhances soups, stews, and grilled meats; also used for color in dishes like deviled eggs.

3. **Turmeric**
    - **Flavor**: Earthy and slightly bitter.

- - Uses: Common in Indian and Southeast Asian dishes, adds vibrant color to curries, rice, and roasted vegetables.
4. **Coriander (Seeds)**
   - **Flavor**: Citrusy and slightly spicy.
   - **Uses**: Ground seeds are used in curries, pickling, and spice blends.
5. **Cinnamon**
   - **Flavor**: Sweet and warm.
   - **Uses**: Adds depth to both sweet and savory dishes, including desserts, stews, and Moroccan tagines.
6. **Ginger**
   - **Flavor**: Spicy and slightly sweet.
   - **Uses**: Fresh or ground, enhances stir-fries, marinades, and baked goods.
7. **Nutmeg**
   - **Flavor**: Warm and nutty.
   - **Uses**: Adds richness to creamy sauces, vegetables, and baked goods like pies and custards.
8. **Chili Powder**
   - **Flavor**: Spicy and smoky.
   - **Uses**: Essential in Tex-Mex cuisine, adds heat to chili, tacos, and marinades.

Tips for Using Herbs and Spices

1. **Fresh vs. Dried**
   - **Fresh Herbs**: Add at the end of cooking or as a garnish to retain their fresh flavors.
   - **Dried Herbs**: Add earlier in cooking to allow flavors to meld; use smaller amounts as they are more concentrated.
2. **Combining Flavors**
   - **Pairing**: Experiment with complementary flavors; for example, rosemary with garlic, or cumin with coriander.
   - **Balancing**: Use a variety of herbs and spices to create depth without overpowering the dish.
3. **Toasting Spices**
   - **Enhancement**: Toast whole spices in a dry skillet before grinding to release essential oils and deepen flavors.
4. **Storage**
   - **Fresh Herbs**: Store in the refrigerator wrapped in damp paper towels or upright in a glass of water.
   - **Dried Herbs and Spices**: Keep in airtight containers away from heat and light to maintain freshness.

Example Recipes

1. **Grilled Lemon-Rosemary Chicken**
   - **Ingredients**: Chicken breasts, fresh rosemary, garlic, lemon juice, olive oil.
   - **Preparation**: Marinate chicken in lemon juice, olive oil, minced garlic, and chopped rosemary. Grill until cooked through.
2. **Vegetable Curry with Cumin and Turmeric**
   - **Ingredients**: Mixed vegetables (like cauliflower, carrots, peas), onion, garlic, ginger, curry powder, cumin, turmeric, coconut milk.
   - **Preparation**: Sauté onion, garlic, and ginger in oil. Add vegetables, spices, and coconut milk. Simmer until vegetables are tender.
3. **Quinoa Salad with Fresh Herbs**
   - **Ingredients**: Cooked quinoa, cucumber, cherry tomatoes, red onion, parsley, mint, lemon juice, olive oil.
   - **Preparation**: Combine all ingredients in a bowl. Season with lemon juice, olive oil, salt, and pepper.
4. **Spiced Roasted Sweet Potatoes**
   - **Ingredients**: Sweet potatoes, olive oil, paprika, cinnamon, salt.

- **Preparation**: Toss sweet potatoes with olive oil, paprika, cinnamon, and salt. Roast until tender and caramelized.

Incorporating herbs and spices into meals not only enhances flavor but also reduces the need for added salt, supporting a heart-healthy diet for stroke patients.

Chapter 9

9.1 Importance of Exercise in Recovery

Exercise plays a crucial role in the recovery process for stroke patients, offering numerous physical and psychological benefits. Here's an overview of why exercise is important and how it supports recovery:

Importance of Exercise in Recovery from Stroke

1. **Physical Rehabilitation**
   - **Motor Skills**: Helps regain and improve motor skills, including walking, balance, and coordination.
   - **Strength**: Builds muscle strength and endurance, which may have been weakened due to stroke-related immobility.
   - **Flexibility**: Improves flexibility and range of motion in affected limbs.
2. **Cardiovascular Health**
   - **Heart Health**: Reduces the risk of cardiovascular diseases, which are common after stroke.
   - **Blood Circulation**: Enhances blood circulation and oxygen delivery to the brain and body tissues, supporting overall recovery.

3. **Prevention of Secondary Complications**
   - **Muscle Atrophy**: Counteracts muscle atrophy and stiffness, preventing contractures (permanent shortening of muscles).
   - **Joint Health**: Maintains joint health and reduces the risk of joint pain and stiffness.
4. **Mental and Emotional Well-being**
   - **Mood Improvement**: Releases endorphins that improve mood and reduce feelings of depression and anxiety.
   - **Self-Esteem**: Boosts self-esteem and confidence as patients regain physical abilities and independence.
   - **Cognitive Function**: Supports cognitive function and enhances overall mental alertness and clarity.
5. **Stroke Risk Reduction**
   - **Secondary Stroke**: Reduces the risk of recurrent strokes by promoting heart health and managing related risk factors like hypertension and diabetes.
6. **Social Interaction**
   - **Support Network**: Provides opportunities for social interaction and engagement through group exercise classes or therapy sessions.

Types of Recommended Exercises

1. **Physical Therapy Exercises**
    - **Range of Motion**: Includes passive and active exercises to improve flexibility and movement in affected limbs.
    - **Strength Training**: Uses resistance exercises to build muscle strength and endurance.
    - **Balance and Coordination**: Focuses on exercises to improve balance and coordination, reducing the risk of falls.
2. **Aerobic Exercises**
    - **Walking**: Gradually increasing walking distance and speed.
    - **Stationary Cycling**: Low-impact exercise that improves cardiovascular fitness.
    - **Swimming**: Provides a full-body workout with low joint impact.
3. **Activities of Daily Living (ADL) Exercises**
    - **Functional Training**: Integrates exercises that mimic daily tasks to improve independence in self-care activities.
4. **Adaptive and Assistive Devices**
    - **Supportive Equipment**: Uses devices like walkers, canes, or orthoses to assist with mobility and exercises.

Considerations for Stroke Patients

1. **Individualized Plans**
   - **Rehabilitation Team**: Works with a multidisciplinary team to create personalized exercise plans based on the patient's abilities and goals.
   - **Progress Monitoring**: Adjusts exercises as recovery progresses to ensure continued improvement.

2. **Safety Precautions**
   - **Supervision**: Exercises should be supervised initially to ensure safety and proper technique.
   - **Warm-up and Cool-down**: Includes proper warm-up and cool-down routines to prevent injury and manage fatigue.

3. **Consistency and Persistence**
   - **Routine**: Establishes a regular exercise routine to maximize benefits and maintain long-term health.
   - **Motivation**: Encourages ongoing participation through positive reinforcement and goal setting.

Exercise plays a pivotal role in stroke recovery, offering physical, mental, and emotional benefits that contribute to overall well-being. By incorporating appropriate exercises tailored to individual needs and capabilities, stroke patients can enhance their recovery, regain functional abilities, and improve their quality of life. Regular consultation with healthcare providers ensures safe and effective exercise participation throughout the recovery journey.

9.2 Safe Exercises for Stroke Patients

Safe and appropriate exercises are crucial for stroke patients to aid in their recovery without compromising their health or safety. Here's a guide to safe exercises tailored for stroke patients, focusing on improving mobility, strength, balance, and overall well-being:

Safe Exercises for Stroke Patients

1. Range of Motion Exercises

- **Description**: These exercises aim to improve flexibility and joint mobility, crucial for preventing muscle stiffness and contractures.
- **Examples**: Gentle stretching of arms, legs, and neck. Passive range of motion exercises with assistance from a caregiver or physical therapist.

2. Strength Training

- **Description**: Building strength helps regain muscle mass lost due to stroke-induced immobility, supporting better functional movement.
- **Examples**:
  - **Upper Body**: Arm curls with light weights or resistance bands.
  - **Lower Body**: Leg lifts while seated or standing with support.
  - **Core**: Pelvic tilts and gentle abdominal crunches.

3. Balance and Coordination Exercises

- **Description**: Enhancing balance reduces the risk of falls and improves overall stability.
- **Examples**:
  - **Standing Balance**: Stand near a stable surface and lift one leg for a few seconds, gradually increasing duration.

- o **Weight Shifts**: Shift weight from side to side or forward and backward while standing.

4. Walking and Gait Training

- **Description**: Walking exercises help improve gait patterns and regain mobility.
- **Examples**:
  - o **Assisted Walking**: Use of a cane, walker, or physical assistance initially.
  - o **Treadmill Training**: Under supervision to improve walking speed and endurance.

5. Aerobic Exercises

- **Description**: Cardiovascular exercises improve heart health and overall stamina.
- **Examples**:
  - o **Stationary Cycling**: Low-impact option to improve leg strength and cardiovascular endurance.
  - o **Water Aerobics**: Provides buoyancy and reduces impact on joints while improving cardiovascular fitness.

6. Functional Activities

- **Description**: Practicing daily tasks helps regain independence in activities of daily living (ADLs).
- **Examples**:
  - **Dressing**: Practice putting on clothes with affected limbs.
  - **Cooking**: Engage in simple cooking tasks to improve coordination and dexterity.

7. Yoga and Tai Chi

- **Description**: These activities combine gentle movements, breathing exercises, and mindfulness, promoting relaxation and flexibility.
- **Examples**: Modified yoga poses and Tai Chi movements focusing on balance and gentle stretching.

8. Speech and Swallowing Exercises

- **Description**: For stroke patients with speech and swallowing difficulties (dysphagia), specific exercises can help improve these functions.
- **Examples**: Tongue exercises, swallowing techniques, and vocalization exercises under the guidance of a speech therapist.

Considerations for Safety

- **Consultation**: Always consult with a healthcare professional or physical therapist before starting any exercise program.
- **Gradual Progression**: Start with low-intensity exercises and gradually increase intensity and duration as tolerance improves.
- **Monitoring**: Exercise should be supervised, especially initially, to ensure safety and proper technique.
- **Adaptations**: Modify exercises based on individual abilities and limitations to prevent injury.
- **Hydration and Rest**: Stay hydrated and take breaks as needed during exercise sessions.

Incorporating these safe exercises into a comprehensive rehabilitation plan can greatly benefit stroke patients by improving physical function, enhancing quality of life, and promoting independence. Regular assessment and adjustments by healthcare professionals ensure that exercise programs remain safe and effective throughout the recovery journey.

9.3 Combining Diet and Exercise for Better Health

Combining a healthy diet with regular exercise is essential for achieving and maintaining better health, especially for stroke patients who are focused on recovery and overall well-being. Here's how integrating both components can synergistically enhance health outcomes:

Benefits of Combining Diet and Exercise

1. **Weight Management**
   - **Diet**: A balanced diet rich in fruits, vegetables, lean proteins, and whole grains helps control calorie intake.
   - **Exercise**: Regular physical activity, such as aerobic exercises and strength training, burns calories and supports weight loss or maintenance.
2. **Cardiovascular Health**
   - **Diet**: Low-sodium, heart-healthy foods reduce blood pressure and cholesterol levels.
   - **Exercise**: Aerobic exercises like walking, swimming, or cycling strengthen the heart and improve circulation.

3. **Muscle Strength and Mobility**
   - **Diet**: Protein-rich foods support muscle repair and growth.
   - **Exercise**: Strength training exercises enhance muscle strength, flexibility, and coordination, crucial for mobility and daily activities.
4. **Mental Well-being**
   - **Diet**: Nutrient-dense foods, including omega-3 fatty acids and antioxidants, support brain health and mood stability.
   - **Exercise**: Releases endorphins that reduce stress, anxiety, and symptoms of depression, promoting mental clarity and well-being.
5. **Energy Levels**
   - **Diet**: Balanced meals with complex carbohydrates provide sustained energy throughout the day.
   - **Exercise**: Boosts energy levels and reduces fatigue by improving cardiovascular efficiency and overall fitness.
6. **Bone Health**
   - **Diet**: Calcium-rich foods and vitamin D support bone strength and density.
   - **Exercise**: Weight-bearing exercises, such as walking or dancing, help

maintain bone health and reduce the risk of osteoporosis.

Tips for Integrating Diet and Exercise

1. **Consultation with Healthcare Professionals**
   - **Individualized Plan**: Work with a dietitian and physical therapist to create personalized diet and exercise plans tailored to specific health needs and goals.
2. **Balanced Nutrition**
   - **Healthy Choices**: Include a variety of fruits, vegetables, whole grains, lean proteins, and healthy fats in your diet.
   - **Portion Control**: Practice mindful eating and control portion sizes to manage calorie intake effectively.
3. **Regular Physical Activity**
   - **Routine**: Establish a regular exercise routine that includes aerobic exercises, strength training, flexibility exercises, and balance training.
   - **Consistency**: Aim for at least 150 minutes of moderate-intensity aerobic activity per week, along with muscle-strengthening exercises on two or more days per week.
4. **Hydration**

- o **Importance**: Drink an adequate amount of water throughout the day to stay hydrated, support digestion, and maintain overall health.

5. **Monitor Progress**
   - o **Tracking**: Keep a record of dietary intake and exercise sessions to monitor progress and make adjustments as needed.
   - o **Feedback**: Regularly review progress with healthcare professionals to ensure goals are being met and adjust plans accordingly.

Example of a Combined Approach

- **Breakfast**: Whole grain oats with berries and a sprinkle of nuts or seeds.
- **Lunch**: Grilled chicken salad with mixed greens, tomatoes, cucumbers, and a light vinaigrette.
- **Dinner**: Baked salmon with quinoa and steamed vegetables.
- **Snacks**: Greek yogurt with fruit, or carrot sticks with hummus.
- **Exercise**: Morning walk or cycling for 30 minutes, followed by light strength training exercises targeting major muscle groups.

By integrating a nutritious diet with regular physical activity, stroke patients can optimize their recovery, improve overall health, and reduce the risk of future health complications. Consistency, moderation, and personalized guidance from healthcare professionals are key to achieving sustainable health benefits.

Chapter 10

10.1 Finding Support Groups

Finding support groups can be invaluable for stroke patients and their caregivers, providing emotional support, information sharing, and opportunities to connect with others facing similar challenges. Here are some ways to find support groups:

Finding Support Groups for Stroke Patients

1. **Hospitals and Rehabilitation Centers**
   - Many hospitals and rehabilitation centers offer support groups specifically for stroke patients and their families.
   - **How to Find**: Inquire with your healthcare provider or rehabilitation team during hospital visits or outpatient appointments.
2. **Local Community Centers**
   - Community centers often host support groups for various health conditions, including stroke.
   - **How to Find**: Contact local community centers or check their websites for information on health-related support groups.

3. **Online Resources and Forums**
   - Online platforms and forums provide virtual support groups where individuals can connect from anywhere.
   - **Examples**: Websites like Stroke Support Association, American Stroke Association's Support Network, or social media groups dedicated to stroke recovery.
4. **Nonprofit Organizations**
   - Organizations focused on stroke recovery often facilitate support groups and provide resources for patients and caregivers.
   - **Examples**: American Heart Association, National Stroke Association, or local nonprofit organizations dedicated to stroke awareness and support.

5. **Social Media and Apps**
   - Social media platforms and apps may host groups or forums where stroke survivors and caregivers share experiences and offer support.

- o **Examples**: Facebook groups, Reddit communities, or specialized apps for health support.

6. **Healthcare Provider Referrals**
   - o Your primary care physician, neurologist, or rehabilitation specialist can recommend local support groups or online resources.
   - o **How to Find**: Ask your healthcare provider during appointments or consultations.

7. **Stroke Rehabilitation Programs**
   - o Rehabilitation programs often include group therapy sessions or support groups as part of their services.
   - o **How to Find**: Inquire with your rehabilitation therapist or coordinator about available support group options.

8. **National Stroke Associations**
   - o National stroke associations often maintain directories or databases of local support groups and resources.
   - o **Examples**: Check websites of organizations like the American Stroke Association or Stroke Foundation in your country.

Tips for Choosing a Support Group

- **Accessibility**: Choose a support group that is accessible in terms of location (if in-person) or online platform (if virtual).
- **Size and Format**: Consider whether you prefer smaller, intimate groups or larger gatherings, as well as the format (in-person, virtual, or both).
- **Focus**: Some groups may focus on specific aspects of stroke recovery, such as physical rehabilitation, emotional support, or caregiving challenges.
- **Frequency**: Check the meeting frequency and schedule that fits your availability and needs.
- **Comfort Level**: Attend a meeting or session to gauge the comfort level, group dynamics, and whether it meets your expectations.

Finding a support group for stroke patients and caregivers can provide valuable emotional support, information sharing, and a sense of community during the recovery journey. Explore various options, both in-person and online, to find a support group that meets your specific needs and preferences. Support groups can offer encouragement, practical advice, and a shared understanding of the challenges and triumphs associated with stroke recovery.

10.2 Online Resources and Apps

There are several online resources and apps specifically designed to support stroke patients and their caregivers. These platforms provide information, tools, and communities where individuals can find guidance, connect with others, and access resources related to stroke recovery. Here are some notable online resources and apps:

Online Resources for Stroke Patients

1. **American Stroke Association**
   - Website: American Stroke Association
   - **Features**: Offers information on stroke prevention, recovery, and support resources. Includes access to their Support Network for connecting with others affected by stroke.
2. **National Stroke Association**
   - Website: National Stroke Association
   - **Features**: Provides education, resources, and support for stroke

survivors, caregivers, and healthcare professionals. Includes information on recovery, advocacy, and community events.

3. **World Stroke Organization**
   - Website: World Stroke Organization
   - **Features**: Global organization dedicated to stroke prevention, treatment, and support. Offers resources, educational materials, and information on research and advocacy efforts.

4. **Stroke Support Association**
   - Website: Stroke Support Association
   - **Features**: Provides support groups, educational programs, and resources for stroke survivors and caregivers in Southern California. Offers online resources and virtual support options.

5. **HealthUnlocked**
   - Website: HealthUnlocked
   - **Features**: Online community platform where individuals can join health-related forums, including stroke recovery and support groups. Offers peer support and information sharing.

Mobile Apps for Stroke Recovery

1. **MyHeartCounts**

- **Platform**: iOS
- **Features**: Developed by Stanford Medicine, focuses on heart health but includes resources and tracking tools useful for stroke patients managing cardiovascular health.

2. **American Heart Association's Heart360**
   - **Platform**: iOS, Android
   - **Features**: Tracks blood pressure, cholesterol, and other health metrics relevant to stroke prevention and management. Provides educational resources and goal setting.

3. **Stroke Support**
   - **Platform**: iOS
   - **Features**: Provides information on stroke signs, symptoms, and recovery. Includes tools for tracking progress, medication reminders, and connecting with support networks.

4. **Neuro Rehab VR**
   - **Platform**: Oculus VR
   - **Features**: Virtual reality therapy designed for stroke rehabilitation, offering immersive exercises to improve motor skills and cognitive functions.

5. **Brain Exercise with Dr. Kawashima**
   - **Platform**: iOS, Android

- o **Features**: Brain training app with games and exercises designed to improve cognitive functions such as memory and attention, which can be beneficial for stroke recovery.

Tips for Using Online Resources and Apps

- **Research**: Explore different resources and apps to find those that best suit your needs and preferences.
- **User Reviews**: Check user reviews and ratings to gauge the effectiveness and usability of apps.
- **Accessibility**: Ensure the app or website is accessible and user-friendly for your specific requirements.
- **Privacy**: Review privacy policies and ensure your personal information is protected when using apps or joining online communities.

Utilizing online resources and apps can complement traditional healthcare support for stroke patients and caregivers, providing convenient access to information, tools for tracking progress, and communities for support and encouragement. Whether seeking educational materials, tracking health metrics, or connecting with others in similar situations, these resources can enhance the stroke recovery journey and promote overall well-being.

10.3 Working with Dietitians and Nutritionists

Working with dietitians and nutritionists can be highly beneficial for stroke patients and their caregivers, as they play a crucial role in developing personalized dietary plans that support recovery, promote overall health, and reduce the risk of future health complications. Here's how dietitians and nutritionists can help:

Role of Dietitians and Nutritionists in Stroke Recovery

1. **Assessment and Personalized Nutrition Plans**
   - **Evaluation**: Conduct a thorough assessment of the patient's medical history, current health status, nutritional needs, and dietary preferences.

- **Customized Plans**: Develop personalized nutrition plans tailored to meet specific health goals, such as managing blood pressure, cholesterol levels, and weight.

2. **Education and Nutritional Guidance**
   - **Education**: Provide evidence-based information on the importance of nutrition in stroke recovery and prevention.
   - **Guidance**: Offer practical guidance on portion control, food choices, and meal planning to support a balanced diet.

3. **Managing Special Dietary Needs**
   - **Dietary Restrictions**: Address specific dietary restrictions or concerns, such as allergies, food intolerances, or dysphagia (swallowing difficulties).
   - **Nutrient Requirements**: Ensure adequate intake of essential nutrients, vitamins, and minerals necessary for recovery and overall health.

4. **Monitoring and Support**
   - **Progress Monitoring**: Track dietary habits and nutritional status to assess progress and make adjustments as needed.

- o **Continuous Support**: Provide ongoing support, motivation, and accountability to help patients adhere to dietary recommendations and achieve health goals.

5. **Collaboration with Healthcare Team**
   - o **Multidisciplinary Approach**: Work collaboratively with physicians, therapists, and other healthcare professionals to integrate nutrition therapy into comprehensive stroke rehabilitation programs.
   - o **Coordination**: Ensure continuity of care and communication regarding dietary changes and their impact on overall health and recovery.

Tips for Working Effectively with Dietitians and Nutritionists

- **Open Communication**: Share concerns, preferences, and any challenges related to dietary changes openly with your dietitian or nutritionist.
- **Follow Recommendations**: Adhere to dietary recommendations and guidelines provided by your healthcare team to maximize benefits.
- **Ask Questions**: Seek clarification on nutrition-related information or

recommendations to enhance understanding and compliance.

- **Keep Records**: Maintain a food diary or record dietary intake to facilitate discussions and adjustments during consultations.
- **Stay Engaged**: Actively participate in nutrition counseling sessions, ask for resources, and stay informed about dietary strategies for stroke recovery.

Dietitians and nutritionists play a pivotal role in supporting stroke patients by providing personalized nutrition plans, education, and ongoing guidance to optimize recovery and promote overall health. Their expertise in dietary management and collaborative approach with healthcare professionals contribute significantly to the holistic care and well-being of stroke survivors and their caregivers. Working closely with a qualified dietitian or nutritionist can empower individuals to make informed dietary choices and achieve long-term health goals after stroke.

Chapter 11

11.1 Long-term Dietary Habits

Long-term dietary habits are crucial for stroke patients to maintain overall health, manage risk factors, and support ongoing recovery. Establishing healthy eating habits can help prevent complications and promote well-being over the long term. Here are key considerations for developing and maintaining beneficial dietary habits after a stroke:

Key Principles for Long-Term Dietary Habits

1. **Balanced Nutrition**
   - **Variety**: Include a variety of fruits, vegetables, whole grains, lean proteins (such as poultry, fish, beans, and legumes), and healthy fats (such as nuts, seeds, and olive oil) in your diet.
   - **Portion Control**: Monitor portion sizes to manage calorie intake and maintain a healthy weight.

2. **Heart-Healthy Eating**

- **Reduce Saturated Fat**: Limit intake of foods high in saturated fats, such as fatty meats, full-fat dairy products, and processed foods.
- **Increase Omega-3 Fatty Acids**: Incorporate sources of omega-3 fatty acids, such as fatty fish (salmon, mackerel, sardines), flaxseeds, and walnuts, which support heart health.

3. **Low Sodium Intake**
   - **Limit Salt**: Reduce salt intake to lower blood pressure and manage fluid retention. Use herbs, spices, and citrus juices to flavor foods instead of salt.
   - **Read Labels**: Check food labels for sodium content and choose low-sodium or no-added-salt options whenever possible.

4. **Fiber-Rich Foods**
   - **Whole Grains**: Opt for whole grains like brown rice, whole wheat bread, oats, and quinoa, which provide fiber to support digestive health and regulate blood sugar levels.
   - **Fruits and Vegetables**: Eat a variety of colorful fruits and vegetables daily to increase fiber intake and benefit from essential vitamins and minerals.

5. **Hydration**

- **Water**: Drink plenty of water throughout the day to stay hydrated, support digestion, and maintain overall health.
  - **Limit Sugary Drinks**: Reduce consumption of sugary beverages and opt for water, herbal teas, or infused water for hydration.

6. **Monitoring and Moderation**
   - **Keep Track**: Maintain a food diary or use a mobile app to track dietary habits and monitor progress towards health goals.
   - **Moderation**: Enjoy treats and less healthy foods occasionally in moderation, while focusing on a predominantly nutritious diet.

7. **Consistency and Routine**
   - **Regular Meals**: Establish regular eating patterns with balanced meals and healthy snacks to maintain energy levels and support metabolism.
   - **Meal Planning**: Plan meals ahead to ensure nutritious choices and avoid impulsive or unhealthy eating habits.

8. **Lifestyle and Mindful Eating**
   - **Physical Activity**: Combine a healthy diet with regular physical activity to enhance cardiovascular health,

manage weight, and improve overall well-being.
  - **Mindful Eating**: Practice mindful eating by paying attention to hunger and fullness cues, savoring flavors, and avoiding distractions during meals.

Collaborative Approach

- **Healthcare Team**: Work closely with your healthcare team, including dietitians, physicians, and therapists, to develop and adjust dietary plans based on individual health needs and recovery goals.
- **Support Network**: Engage with support groups, family members, and caregivers to maintain motivation, share experiences, and seek guidance on long-term dietary habits.

Long-term dietary habits play a critical role in supporting stroke recovery and overall health. By adopting a balanced, heart-healthy diet rich in nutrients and low in sodium, individuals can manage risk factors, enhance physical well-being, and promote longevity. Consistency, moderation, and collaboration with healthcare professionals are key to sustaining beneficial dietary habits over time.

11.2 Maintaining a Healthy Lifestyle Post-Recovery

Maintaining a healthy lifestyle post-recovery from a stroke is crucial for preventing recurrence, managing ongoing health issues, and promoting overall well-being. Here are essential aspects to consider for maintaining a healthy lifestyle after stroke:

1. Healthy Eating Habits

- **Balanced Diet**: Continue to prioritize a balanced diet rich in fruits, vegetables, whole grains, lean proteins, and healthy fats.
- **Portion Control**: Monitor portion sizes to manage weight and prevent overeating.
- **Limit Sodium and Saturated Fats**: Reduce intake of salt and foods high in saturated fats to support heart health.
- **Hydration**: Drink plenty of water throughout the day to stay hydrated and support bodily functions.
- **Regular Meals**: Maintain regular meal times to stabilize blood sugar levels and energy throughout the day.

2. Regular Physical Activity

- **Aerobic Exercise**: Engage in regular aerobic activities such as walking, cycling, or swimming to improve cardiovascular health and endurance.
- **Strength Training**: Incorporate strength training exercises to build muscle strength and support mobility.
- **Flexibility and Balance**: Practice activities like yoga or tai chi to improve flexibility, balance, and reduce the risk of falls.
- **Moderation and Consistency**: Aim for at least 150 minutes of moderate-intensity aerobic activity per week, spread throughout the week.

3. Manage Risk Factors

- **Blood Pressure Control**: Monitor and manage blood pressure levels with the help of healthcare professionals.
- **Cholesterol Management**: Maintain healthy cholesterol levels through diet, exercise, and medication as prescribed.
- **Blood Sugar Regulation**: Manage diabetes or prediabetes through diet, exercise, and medication under medical supervision.

- **Quit Smoking**: If applicable, quit smoking to reduce the risk of further cardiovascular complications.

4. Stress Management and Mental Well-being

- **Mindfulness and Relaxation Techniques**: Practice mindfulness, deep breathing exercises, or meditation to reduce stress and promote relaxation.
- **Social Engagement**: Stay connected with friends, family, and support groups to maintain social connections and emotional well-being.
- **Seek Support**: Don't hesitate to seek professional help from counselors or therapists for emotional support and coping strategies.

5. Regular Health Monitoring

- **Medical Check-ups**: Attend regular follow-up appointments with healthcare providers to monitor health status, medications, and make necessary adjustments.
- **Screenings**: Schedule recommended screenings for cardiovascular health, diabetes, and other relevant conditions based on healthcare provider recommendations.

6. Maintain Cognitive Function

- **Brain Exercises**: Stay mentally active with puzzles, reading, learning new skills, or brain-training exercises to maintain cognitive function.
- **Sleep**: Aim for adequate and quality sleep to support brain health and overall well-being.

7. Adopting a Positive Mindset

- **Setting Realistic Goals**: Set achievable goals for health improvement and celebrate progress along the way.
- **Stay Motivated**: Stay motivated by focusing on the benefits of a healthy lifestyle and the positive impact on overall quality of life.
- **Adaptability**: Be open to adapting routines and habits as needed to maintain long-term health and well-being.

Maintaining a healthy lifestyle post-recovery from stroke requires a holistic approach that includes healthy eating habits, regular physical activity, managing risk factors, addressing mental well-being, regular health monitoring, and adopting a positive mindset. By incorporating these elements into daily life and working closely with healthcare professionals, individuals can enhance their recovery, reduce the risk of future health issues, and improve overall quality of life after stroke.

Chapter 12

12.1 Sample Meal Plans

Creating sample meal plans for stroke patients focuses on nutrient-dense foods that support recovery, manage risk factors like high blood pressure and cholesterol, and promote overall health. Here are examples of balanced meal plans for breakfast, lunch, and dinner:

Sample Meal Plans for Stroke Patients

Breakfast

Option 1: Oatmeal with Berries and Nuts

- **Ingredients**:
    1. 1/2 cup of rolled oats
    2. 1 cup of skim milk or almond milk
    3. 1/2 cup of mixed berries (such as blueberries, strawberries)
    4. 1 tablespoon of chopped nuts (almonds, walnuts)
    5. 1 teaspoon of honey or maple syrup (optional)
- **Instructions**:
    1. Cook oats with milk according to package instructions.

2. Top with berries, nuts, and a drizzle of honey or maple syrup.
3. Serve warm.

Option 2: Greek Yogurt Parfait

- **Ingredients**:
    1. 1/2 cup of Greek yogurt (plain, low-fat)
    2. 1/4 cup of granola (low-sugar)
    3. 1/2 cup of mixed fresh fruits (such as bananas, apples, kiwi)
    4. 1 tablespoon of chia seeds or flaxseeds
- **Instructions**:
    1. Layer yogurt, granola, and fruits in a bowl or parfait glass.
    2. Sprinkle with chia seeds or flaxseeds.
    3. Enjoy chilled.

Lunch

Option 1: Grilled Chicken Salad

- **Ingredients**:
    1. 3 oz. grilled chicken breast, sliced
    2. Mixed greens (spinach, arugula)
    3. 1/2 cup of cherry tomatoes, halved
    4. 1/4 cucumber, sliced
    5. 1/4 avocado, sliced

6. 1 tablespoon of olive oil and balsamic vinegar dressing

- **Instructions**:
    1. Arrange mixed greens on a plate.
    2. Top with grilled chicken, cherry tomatoes, cucumber, and avocado.
    3. Drizzle with olive oil and balsamic vinegar dressing.

Option 2: Quinoa and Vegetable Stir-fry

- **Ingredients**:
    1. 1/2 cup of quinoa, cooked
    2. 1 cup of mixed vegetables (bell peppers, broccoli, carrots)
    3. 3 oz. of tofu or lean protein (chicken, shrimp)
    4. 1 tablespoon of low-sodium soy sauce
    5. 1 teaspoon of sesame oil
    6. Sprinkle of sesame seeds
- **Instructions**:
    1. Heat sesame oil in a pan and stir-fry tofu or protein until cooked.
    2. Add mixed vegetables and cook until tender-crisp.
    3. Stir in cooked quinoa and soy sauce, toss to combine.
    4. Garnish with sesame seeds and serve.

Dinner

Option 1: Baked Salmon with Quinoa and Steamed Vegetables

- **Ingredients**:
    1. 4 oz. salmon fillet, seasoned with lemon and herbs
    2. 1/2 cup of quinoa, cooked
    3. Steamed vegetables (broccoli, carrots)
- **Instructions**:
    1. Preheat oven to 375°F (190°C).
    2. Place seasoned salmon on a baking sheet and bake for 15-20 minutes until cooked through.
    3. Serve with quinoa and steamed vegetables.

Option 2: Turkey and Vegetable Stir-fry with Brown Rice

- **Ingredients**:
    1. 3 oz. lean turkey breast, sliced
    2. 1 cup of mixed vegetables (snow peas, bell peppers, mushrooms)
    3. 1/2 cup of cooked brown rice
    4. 1 tablespoon of low-sodium teriyaki sauce
- **Instructions**:
    1. Heat a non-stick skillet over medium heat and cook turkey until browned and cooked through.

2. Add mixed vegetables and stir-fry until tender-crisp.
3. Stir in cooked brown rice and teriyaki sauce, cook until heated through.
4. Serve hot.

Tips for Meal Planning:

- **Nutrient Density**: Include a variety of colors in fruits and vegetables to ensure a range of nutrients.
- **Lean Proteins**: Choose lean proteins such as poultry, fish, tofu, or legumes for heart health.
- **Healthy Fats**: Incorporate sources of healthy fats like olive oil, nuts, seeds, and avocado in moderation.
- **Whole Grains**: Opt for whole grains such as quinoa, brown rice, and oats for fiber and sustained energy.
- **Hydration**: Pair meals with water or herbal teas to stay hydrated throughout the day.

These sample meal plans provide a foundation for balanced nutrition tailored to support recovery and maintain health post-stroke. Adjust portions and ingredients based on individual dietary needs and preferences, and consult with a healthcare provider or dietitian for personalized recommendations.

www.ingramcontent.com/pod-product-compliance
Lightning Source LLC
Chambersburg PA
CBHW061632250726

48659CB00004B/1177